American Pharmaceutical Asso(
Basic Pharmacy and Pharmacology Series

MW00977538

Pharmacy Technician

WORKBOOK AND REVIEW

-UPDATE EDITION-

PERSPECTIVE PRESS
MORTON PUBLISHING COMPANY
www.morton-pub.com

Morton Publishing

Printed in the United States of America.

Morton Publishing Company
925 West Kenyon Avenue, Unit 12
Englewood, CO 80110
phone: 1-303-761-4805
fax: 1-303-762-9923

02 03 04 / 9 8 7 6 5 4 3 2

PHARMACY TECHNICIAN

WORKBOOK AND REVIEW

TABLE OF CONTENTS

TABLE OF CONTENTS

ACKNOWLEDGEMENTS

Joe Medina, C.Ph.T., B.S. Pharmacy

Joe Medina contributed to this Workbook and Review by writing many of the exam review questions and other exercises and by helping in the development of the text which this workbook accompanies: **The Pharmacy Technician**, by Perspective Press and Morton Publishing. Joe has served as the Chairperson/Program Director for the Pharmacy Technician Programs at Front Range Community College and Arapahoe Community College in the Denver metro area and has fifteen years experience as a pharmacy technician and twelve years experience as a pharmacist. He also has an Internet business called Tech Lectures® (www.techlectures.com) which strives to not only provide quality continuing education at an affordable price for the pharmacy technician, but more importantly, tries to promote the pharmacy technician profession.

Mary F. Powers, Ph.D., R.Ph.

Mary Powers contributed to this Workbook and Review by writing many of the exam review questions and by helping in the development of the text which this workbook accompanies. Mary is the Coordinator for Pharmacy Technology at Mercy College of Northwest Ohio, Toledo OH. She is also co-author of a **Pharmacy Calculations** text that is an ideal companion to this Workbook and **The Pharmacy Technician**.

Others We'd Like To Thank

This workbook would also not have been possible without the efforts of a large number of people on the text on which it is based, **The Pharmacy Technician**. I'd like to thank them again for their contributions to that book and mention them as well. We couldn't have done it without their help:

Robert P. Shrewsbury, Ph.D., R.Ph., Associate Professor of Pharmaceutics, University of North Carolina-Chapel Hill; Brenda Hanneson Vonderau, B.Sc. (Pharm.), and Peter Vonderau, R.Ph.; Cindy Johnson, R.PH., MSW, Adjunct Faculty, Arapahoe Community College; Andrew Cordiale, CPhT, Hospital Inventory Technician/Buyer; Betsy A. Gilman, Pharm.D.; Pamela Nicoski, Pharm.D., and Elizabeth Dodds, Pharm.D.; Samuel Blackman, M.D., University of Illinois at Chicago Circle, College of Medicine; Janet Wakelin, Director, Pharmacy Technology Program, Cuyahoga Community College, Cleveland OH; Jack Arthur, R.Ph.; Ami Teague Deaton and Lori Coleman of UNC-Chapel Hill; Lynette De Rosa; Robin Cavallo, Pottstown Memorial Medical Center; Tammy Newnam, Claudette Barjoud, and Anna Veltfort; and Doug Morton, whose sponsorship makes this book possible. Finally, I'd like to thank my family whose support and patience is essential and deeply appreciated: Joan, Hannah, Joan, Wilma Jean, and Jimmy.

—Dennis Hogan, Publisher
Perspective Series

PREFACE

THIS WORKBOOK

This workbook was developed to correspond with the textbook, **The Pharmacy Technician** by Perspective Press. For pharmacy technician students, it is a valuable tool for success in your training course. It provides a useful format for memorizing important information and for checking your knowledge of it. Key concepts and terms are carefully explained, and there are over 800 exercises and problems to test your knowledge. Working these exercises out successfully will help you to succeed in your training.

It is important you follow through the workbook chapter by chapter and try answering the questions before looking up the answers. Once you have completed a chapter, review it and try to memorize the answers to the questions you missed.

A REVIEW GUIDE

The workbook can also be used as a review guide in preparing for the National Pharmacy Technician Certification Examination. All its chapters are important in the taking of the National Exam. However, special attention should be placed on Chapter 6 - Calculations, as the exam will have calculation type problem solving that is often challenging for technicians taking the exam. The method used (ratio & proportion) in this section will solve any calculation problem you come across on the National Certification Examination as well as most problems in the pharmacy setting. A careful review of this workbook will prepare you for much of the national exam. However, some questions on that exam require knowledge gained from practice as a technician. Pharmacy technicians who have work experience in a pharmacy setting will therefore have an advantage in taking the National Exam. As an additional study tool, we have included a practice exam at the back of this book in the same *choose the best answer* format of the national exam.

OVERVIEW: PHARMACY TECHNICIAN CERTIFICATION EXAM

The National Pharmacy Technician Certification Examination was established to allow the certification of technicians. The need for highly qualified pharmacy technicians is increasingly important as pharmacists are relinquishing many dispensing duties for more clinical ones, and the technician is playing a greater role.

Currently the national examination is given by the Pharmacy Technician Certification Board (PTCB) and is offered three times a year in the months of March, July, and November. Applications for the taking of this examination must be made two months prior to the scheduled exam day. The cost of taking this examination is at the time of this writing one-hundred and five dollars.

THE EXAM

The examination contains 125 multiple choice questions which are derived from a data base of several thousand questions. Therefore, examinations given on certain dates are not the same as ones given on a different date. The multiple choice format involves four possible answers with only one answer being the best or most correct. The time limit for taking this examination is three hours.

SCORING OF EXAM

The scoring of the examination is based on the combined average of scores in three functional areas:

1. Assisting the Pharmacist in Serving Patients (64% of Exam)

    Includes activities related to traditional pharmacy prescription dispensing and medication distribution, and collecting and organizing information.

2. Maintaining Medication and Inventory Control Systems (25% of Exam)

    Includes activities related to medication and supply purchasing, inventory control, and preparation and distribution of medications according to approved policies and procedures.

3. Participating in the Administration and Management of Pharmacy Practice (11% of Exam)

    Includes activities related to the administrative process for the pharmacy practice center, including: operations, human resources, facilities and equipment, and information systems.

The combined score range of the exam is 300 to 900 points with a passing of 650 points required.

WHAT YOU NEED TO KNOW FOR THE EXAM

Specific information on examination content is provided in the PTCB's **Candidate Handbook**, which can be downloaded from their site: www.ptcb.org. In general, the examination tests:

➡ *knowledge of the role of the pharmacy technician in the pharmacy (i.e., prescriptions, legal issues, compounding, etc.).* This workbook provides an excellent overview of this area, and for technicians with work experience, your experience on the job should reinforce it.

➡ *knowledge of the most commonly used drugs (including trade and generic names, indications, etc.).* Since the pharmacy technician is not responsible for the consultation of patients, this section is limited in the number of questions presented on the exam. Job experience and Appendix A of this workbook are a good preparation.

➡ *ability to perform common calculations (for a specific dose, for additives in IV solutions, for ml/minute and gtt/minute, etc.).* As a result, it's a good idea to thoroughly study the calculation section of this workbook.

For additional information, contact the PTCB at:

Pharmacy Technician Certification Board
2215 Constitution Avenue, NW
Washington, DC 20037-2985
202-429-7576

—Joe Medina

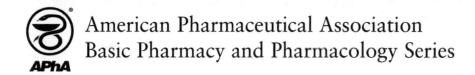

American Pharmaceutical Association
Basic Pharmacy and Pharmacology Series

Dear Student or Instructor,

The American Pharmaceutical Association (APhA), the national professional society of pharmacists in the United States, and Morton Publishing Company, a publisher of educational texts and training materials in healthcare, are pleased to present this outstanding workbook, *Pharmacy Technician Workbook and Review*. It is one of a series of distinctive texts and training materials for basic pharmacy and pharmacology training that is published under this banner: *American Pharmaceutical Association Basic Pharmacy and Pharmacology Series*.

Each book in the series is oriented toward developing an understanding of fundamental concepts. In addition, each text presents applied and practical information on the skills necessary to function effectively in the workplace. Each of the books in the series uses a visual design to enhance understanding and ease of use and is accompanied by various instructional support materials. We think you will find them valuable training tools.

The American Pharmaceutical Association and Morton Publishing thank you for using this book and invite you to look at other titles in this series, which are listed below.

John A. Gans, PharmD
Executive Vice President
American Pharmaceutical Association

Douglas N. Morton
President
Morton Publishing Company

OTHER TITLES IN THIS SERIES:

The Pharmacy Technician
Basic Pharmacology
Drug Card Workbook

NOTICE

To the best of the Publisher's knowledge, the information presented in this book follows general practice as well as federal and state regulations and guidelines. However, please note that you are responsible for following your employer's and your state's policies and guidelines.

The job description for pharmacy technicians varies by institution and state. Your employer and state can provide you with the most recent regulations, guidelines, and practices that apply to your work.

The Publisher of this book disclaims any responsibility whatsoever for any injuries, damages, or other conditions that result from your practice of the skills described in this book for any reason whatsoever.

— 1 —

PHARMACY AND HEALTH CARE

KEY CONCEPTS

Test your knowledge by covering the information in the right hand column.

pharmacology	The study of drugs, their properties, uses, application and effects.
herbal medicine	People have used drugs derived from plants to treat illnesses and other physical conditions for thousands of years. The ancient Greeks used the bark of a white willow tree to relieve pain. The bark contained salicylic acid, the natural forerunner of the active ingredient in aspirin.
cocaine	The first effective local anesthetic.
digitalis	The drug of the foxglove plant which has been widely used in treating heart disease.
quinine	The first useful drug in the treatment of malaria, one of mankind's most deadly diseases. It was extracted from the bark of a Peruvian tree, the Cinchona.
germ theory	The theory that microorganisms cause food spoilage.
pasteurization	The use of heat to kill microorganisms and preserve food, named after Louis Pasteur.
insulin	The hormone that lowers blood sugar in the treatment of diabetes–one of the great discoveries in medicine in the twentieth century.
penicillin	The first antibiotic.

average life span	This measure of health has increased by over twenty years in the United States in the Twentieth Century.
synthetic drugs	Drugs created by reformulating simpler chemicals into more complex ones, creating a new chemical not found in nature.
Human Genome Project	An attempt to map the entire DNA sequence in the human genome. This information will provide a better understanding of hereditary diseases and how to treat them.
pharmacist education and training	In the United States, an individual must graduate from an accredited college of pharmacy, pass a state licensing exam, and perform an internship working under a licensed pharmacist. Once licensed, the pharmacist must receive continuing education to maintain their license.
cost control	A significant trend in recent health care has been the effort to control the cost of prescription drugs, on aspect of which is the use of closed "formularies" that rely substantially on substituting generic drugs in place of more expensive brands.
computerization	Pharmacy computer systems put customer profiles, product, inventory, pricing, and other essential information within easy access. One result has been that pharmacies and pharmacists dispense more prescriptions and information than ever before.

STUDY NOTES

Use this area to write important points you'd like to remember.

FILL IN THE KEY TERM

Use these key terms to fill in the correct blank. Answers are at the end of the book.

antibiotic	hormone	panacea
antitoxin	human genome	Paracelsus
Shen Nung	managed care	pharmaceutical
data	materia medica	pharmacology
formularies	OBRA '90	salicylic acid

1. _____ : an ancient practitioner of "trial and error" drug testing through tasting plants and other natural materials to determine which were poisonous and which were beneficial.

2. _____ : the natural drug derived from the bark of a white willow tree, used by the Ancient Greeks to relieve pain, and the natural forerunner to the active ingredient in aspirin.

3. _____ : an authoritative listing of drugs and issues related to their use.

4. _____ : of or about drugs; also, a drug product.

5. _____ : a cure-all.

6. _____ : the study of drugs—their properties, uses, application, and effects.

7. _____ : he is generally credited with firmly establishing the use of chemistry to create medicinal drugs.

8. _____ : the information stored in a computer.

9. _____ : a substance that acts against a toxin in the body.

10. _____ : a substance which harms or kills microorganisms like bacteria and fungi.

11. _____ : chemicals produced by the body that regulate body functions and processes.

12. _____ : the complete set of genetic material contained in a human cell.

13. _____ : U.S. legislation which required pharmacists to provide consulting services to Medicaid patients.

14. _____ : lists of drugs that are approved for use by patients.

15. _____ : a major factor contributing to the attempt to control costs of prescription drugs.

TRUE/FALSE

Indicate whether the statement is true or false in the blank. Answers are at the end of the book.

_____ 1. The natural drug that is the forerunner to aspirin comes from the cinchona tree.

_____ 2. Almost all drugs used today are made synthetically.

_____ 3. Digitalis comes from the foxglove plant.

_____ 4. Cocaine was the first general anesthetic.

_____ 5. The average life span in the U.S. increased over 50% in the twentieth century.

_____ 6. More pharmacists and technicians are employed in community pharmacies than in any other setting.

_____ 7. The second largest area of employment for pharmacists and technicians is home care.

_____ 8. The pharmacist is generally considered the second most trusted professional, behind doctors.

_____ 9. The use of generic drugs is a major trend in the effort to cut the costs of medication.

_____ 10. Pharmacy computer systems prevent mistakes in data entry.

EXPLAIN WHY

Explain why these statements are true or important. Check your answers in the text. Discuss any questions you may have with your Instructor.

1. Give at least three reasons why synthetic drugs are important.

2. Why was the use of anesthesia revolutionary?

3. Why was Paracelsus's work important?

4. Why was penicillin a major benefit in wartime?

5. Why is the Human Genome Project important to pharmacology?

6. Why are drug patents important?

7. Why are pharmacists among the most trusted professionals?

— 2 —

THE PHARMACY TECHNICIAN

KEY CONCEPTS

Test your knowledge by covering the information in the right hand column.

job responsibilities

Pharmacy technicians perform essential tasks that do not require the pharmacist's skill or expertise. Specific responsibilities and tasks differ by setting and are described in writing by each employer through job descriptions, policy and procedure manuals, and other documents.

supervision

Pharmacy technicians work under the direct supervision of a licensed pharmacist who is legally responsible for their performance.

pharmacist consulting

Having technicians assist the pharmacist frees the pharmacist for activities which require a greater level of expertise, such as consulting with patients.

scope of practice

What individuals may and may not do in their jobs is often referred to as their "scope of practice."

employment opportunities

Like pharmacists, most pharmacy technicians are employed in community pharmacies and hospitals. However, they are also employed in clinics, home care, long term care, mail order prescription pharmacies, and various other settings.

specialized jobs

In various hospital and other environments, there are specialized technician jobs which require more advanced skills developed from additional education, training and experience.

trustworthiness

Pharmacy technicians are entrusted with confidential patient information, dangerous substances, and perishable products.

errors

Drugs, whether prescription or over the counter, can be dangerous if misused, and mistakes by pharmacy technicians can be life-threatening.

math skills
Pharmacy technicians routinely perform mathematical calculations in filling prescriptions and other activities.

terminology
Pharmacy technicians must learn the specific pharmaceutical terminology that will be used on the job.

teamwork
Pharmacy technicians must be able to communicate, cooperate, and work effectively with others.

standards
There is no federal standard for pharmacy technician training or competency. However there are state and employer standards which must be met.

certification
A valuable career step for pharmacy technicians is getting certification by an appropriate organization or body. It verifies an individual's competence as a technician, and indicates a high level of knowledge and skill. In the United States, the Pharmacy Technician Certification Board (PTCB) provides technician national certification.

STUDY NOTES

Use this area to write important points you'd like to remember.

FILL IN THE KEY TERM

Use these key terms to fill in the correct blank. Answers are at the end of the book.

certification   detail oriented   pharmacist
competent   on-the-job training   professionals
confidentiality   patient rights   scope of practice
consulting   patient welfare   technicians
continuing education   personal inventory

1. _____ : what individuals may and may not do in their jobs.

2. _____ : to assess characteristics, skills, qualities, etc.

3. _____ : the requirement of health care providers to keep all patient information private among the patient, the patient's insurer, and the providers directly involved in the patient's care.

4. _____ : the most important consideration in health care.

5. _____ : being qualified and capable to perform a task or job.

6. _____ : a legal proof or document that an individual meets certain objective standards, usually provided by a neutral professional organization.

7. _____ : individuals who are given a basic level of training designed to help them perform specific tasks.

8. _____ : individuals who receive extensive and advanced levels of education before being allowed to practice, such as physicians and pharmacists.

9. _____ : technicians always work under their direct supervision.

10. _____ : one of the services pharmacists provide.

11. _____ : patients are generally guaranteed the right to privacy, confidentiality, the information necessary for informed consent, and the freedom to refuse treatment.

12. _____ : a highly important personal characteristic for technicians, since mistakes with drugs can be life-threatening.

13. _____ : a critical element in maintaining competency for pharmacy technicians.

14. _____ : an important part of training that exposes technicians to workplace settings.

TRUE/FALSE

Indicate whether the statement is true or false in the blank. Answers are at the end of the book.

_____ 1. Specific technician responsibilities differ by setting and job description.

_____ 2. Technicians may sometimes provide consulting services to patients.

_____ 3. Technicians are not allowed to do any work that might have serious consequences for patients.

_____ 4. Mathematics skills are very important to the pharmacy technician.

_____ 5. It is essential for technicians to have good interpersonal skills.

_____ 6. The U.S. government sets standards for technician training.

_____ 7. Patient information is considered public information.

_____ 8. Employers monitor the performance and competency of technicians on an ongoing basis.

_____ 9. The ASHP has developed a national model curriculum.

_____ 10. Once earned, the CPhT designation applies for life.

EXPLAIN WHY

Explain why these statements are true or important. Check your answers in the text. Discuss any questions you may have with your Instructor.

1. Give at least two reasons technicians must work under the supervision of a pharmacist.

2. Why is knowing your "scope of practice important?"

3. Why is dependability important?

4. Why should technicians have math skills?

5. Why are interpersonal skills important?

6. Why is certification a good idea for technicians?

7. Why is continuing education valuable for technicians?

— 3 —

DRUG REGULATION AND CONTROL

KEY CONCEPTS

Test your knowledge by covering the information in the right hand column.

Food and Drug Administration	The leading enforcement agency at the federal level for regulations concerning drug products.
Drug Enforcement Administration	The agency which controls the distribution of drugs that may be easily abused.
Food and Drug Act of 1906	Prohibited interstate commerce in adulterated or misbranded food, drinks, and drugs. Government pre-approval of drugs is required.
1938 Food, Drug and Cosmetic (FDC) Act	In response to the fatal poisoning of 107 people, primarily children, by an untested sulfanilamide concoction, this comprehensive law requires new drugs be shown to be safe before marketing.
1951 Durham-Humphrey Amendment	This law defines what drugs require a prescription by a licensed practitioner and requires them to include this legend on the label: "Caution: Federal Law prohibits dispensing without a prescription."
1962 Kefauver-Harris Amendments	Requires drug manufacturers to provide proof of both safety and effectiveness before marketing the drug.
1970 Poison Prevention Packaging Act	Requires child-proof packaging on all controlled and most prescription drugs dispensed by pharmacies.
1970 Controlled Substances Act (CSA)	The CSA classifies drugs that may be easily abused and restricts their distribution. It is enforced by the Drug Enforcement Administration (DEA) within the Justice Department.
1990 Omnibus Budget Reconciliation Act (OBRA)	Among other things, this act required pharmacists to offer counseling to Medicaid patients regarding medications, effectively putting the common practice into law.

1997 FDA Modernization Act	Changed the legend requirement to "Rx only," with a phase in period until February, 2003.
placebos	Inactive substances, not real medications, that are used to test the effectiveness of drugs.
new drugs	All new drugs, whether made domestically or imported, require FDA approval before they can be marketed in the United States.
clinical tests	Tests on proposed new drugs (investigational drugs) are "controlled" by comparing the effect of a proposed drug on one group of patients with the effect of a different treatment on other patients.
blind tests	Patients in a trial are always "blind" to the treatment, i.e, they are not told which control group they are in. In a "double-blind" test, neither the patients nor the physicians know what the medication is.
patent protection	A patent for a new drug gives its manufacturer an exclusive right to market the drug for a specific period of time under a brand name. A drug patent is in effect for 17 years from the date of the drug's discovery. The Hatch-Waxman Act of 1984 provided for up to five year extensions of patent protection to the patent holders to make up for time lost while products went through the FDA approval process.
generics	Once a patent for a brand drug expires, other manufacturers may copy the drug and release it under its pharmaceutical or "generic" name.
labels and labeling	All drugs are required to have clear and accurate information for all labels, inserts, packaging, and so on, but there are different information requirements for various categories of drugs.
prescription drug labels	The minimum requirements on prescription labels for most drugs are as follows: name and address of dispenser, prescription serial number, date of prescription or filling, name of prescriber, name of patient, directions for use, and cautionary statements.
NDC (National Drug Code) number	The number assigned by the manufacturer. The first five digits indicate the manufacturer. The next four indicate the medication, its strength, and dosage form. The last two indicate the package size.

KEY CONCEPTS

Test your knowledge by covering the information in the right hand column.

controlled substances A drug which has the potential to be abused and for which distribution is controlled by one of five "schedules."

control classifications Manufacturers must clearly label controlled drugs with their control classification.

DEA number The number all prescribers of controlled substances are assigned and which must be used on all controlled drug prescriptions. It has two letters followed by seven single-digit numbers, e.g., AB1234563. The following should always be true of a DEA number on a prescription form: if the sum of the first, third and fifth digits is added to twice the sum of the second, fourth, and sixth digits, the total should be a number whose last digit is the same as the last digit of the DEA number.

risks of approved drugs There is always the risk that an approved drug may produce adverse side effects when used on a larger population.

recalls Recalls are, with a few exceptions, voluntary on the part of the manufacturer. There are three classes of recalls: 1.) where there is a strong likelihood that the product will cause serious adverse effects or death; 2.) where a product may cause temporary but reversible adverse effects, or in which there is little likelihood of serious adverse effects; 3.) where a product is not likely to cause adverse effects.

state regulation State boards of pharmacy are responsible for licensing all prescribers and dispensers and administering regulations for the practice of pharmacy in the state.

liability Legal liability means you can be prosecuted for misconduct.

negligence Failing to do something that should or must be done.

CONTROLLED SUBSTANCE SCHEDULES

The five control schedules are as follows*:

Schedule I:
➥ Each drug has a high potential for abuse and no accepted medical use in the United States. It may not be prescribed. Heroin, various opium derivatives, and hallucinogenic substances are included on this schedule.

Schedule II:
➥ Each drug has a high potential for abuse and may lead to physical or psychological dependence, but also has a currently accepted medical use in the United States. Amphetamines, opium, cocaine, methadone, and various opiates are included on this schedule.

Schedule III:
➥ Each drug's potential for abuse is less than those in Schedules I and II and there is a currently accepted medical use in the U.S., but abuse may lead to moderate or low physical dependence or high psychological dependence. Anabolic steroids and various compounds containing limited quantities of narcotic substances such as codeine are included on this schedule.

Schedule IV:
➥ Each drug has a low potential for abuse relative to Schedule III drugs and there is a current accepted medical use in the U.S., but abuse may lead to limited physical dependence or psychological dependence. Phenobarbital, the sedative chloral hydrate, and the anesthetic methohexital are included in this group.

Schedule V:
➥ Each drug has a low potential for abuse relative to Schedule IV drugs and there is a current accepted medical use in the U.S., but abuse may lead to limited physical dependence or psychological dependence. Compounds containing limited amounts of a narcotic such as codeine are included in this group.

*21 USC Sec. 812. Note: these schedules are revised periodically. It is important to refer to the most current schedule.

Controlled-Substance Prescriptions

Controlled-substance prescriptions have greater requirements at both federal and state levels than other prescriptions, particularly Schedule II drugs. On controlled substance prescriptions, the DEA number must appear on the form and the patient's full street address must be entered.

On Schedule II prescriptions, the form must be signed by the prescriber (no phoned or faxed prescriptions allowed). In many states, there are specific time limits that require Schedule II prescriptions be promptly filled.

Quantities are limited and no refills are allowed. When the prescription is filled, the pharmacist draws a line across it indicating it has been filled.

Federal requirements for Schedules III-V are less stringent than for Schedule II. *For example, Schedules III-V prescriptions may be refilled up to five times within six months.* However, state and other regulations may be stricter than federal requirements, so it is necessary to know the requirements for your specific job setting.

FILL IN THE KEY TERM

Use these key terms to fill in the correct blank. Answers are at the end of the book.

adverse effect	legend drug	pediatric
controlled substance mark	liability	placebo
DEA number	"look-alike" regulation	recall
injunction	NDC (National Drug Code)	therapeutic
labeling	negligence	

1. _____ : the number all prescribers of controlled substances are assigned and which must be used on all controlled drug prescriptions.

2. _____ : a court order preventing a specific action, such as the distribution of a potentially dangerous drug.

3. _____ : an inactive substance given in place of a medication.

4. _____ : an unintended side affect of a medication that is negative or in some way injurious to a patient's health.

5. _____ : any drug which requires a prescription and this "legend" on the label: Rx only.

6. _____ : failing to do something you should have done

7. _____ : having to do with the treatment of children.

8. _____ : important associated information that is not on the label of a drug product itself.

9. _____ : Federal laws require that a drug and/or its container not be imitative of another drug so that the consumer will be misled.

10. _____ : means you can be prosecuted for misconduct.

11. _____ : serving to cure or heal.

12. _____ : the action taken to remove a drug from the market and have it returned to the manufacturer.

13. _____ : the mark (CII-CV) which indicates the control category of a drug with a potential for abuse.

14. _____ : the number on a manufacturer's label indicating the manufacturer and product information.

TRUE/FALSE

Indicate whether the statement is true or false in the blank. Answers are at the end of the book.

_____ 1. Child-proof packaging was required by the Fair Packaging and Labeling Act.

_____ 2. Before it is approved for marketing, a new drug must be shown to be risk free.

_____ 3. Only about 25% of drugs tested on humans are approved for use by the FDA.

_____ 4. Over-the-counter medications do not require a prescription but sometimes prescriptions are written for them.

_____ 5. A prescription serial number must appear on the label of a dispensed prescription container.

_____ 6. Manufacturers are allowed to put controlled substance marks and storage requirements on accompanying labeling for their stock products rather than on the label itself.

_____ 7. Schedule II drugs must be stored in a locked tamper-proof narcotics cabinet.

_____ 8. Schedule III, IV, and V drugs may be stored openly on shelves in retail and hospital settings.

_____ 9. All controlled substances must be ordered using a DEA controlled substance order form.

_____ 10. Most recalls are voluntary.

EXPLAIN WHY

Explain why these statements are true or important. Check your answers in the text. Discuss any questions you may have with your Instructor.

1. Why is blind testing used in the drug approval process?

2. Give three reasons why OTC labels should be clear and understandable.

3. Why are some drugs "controlled" by the DEA?

4. Why are some drug patents extended past the original 17 year period.

5. Why would a manufacturer want to recall a drug product?

6. Give three reasons why failing to do something could result in a criminal charge of negligence.

MATCH THE TERM — CONTROLLED SUBSTANCES AND RECALLS

Use these key terms to fill in the correct blank. Answers are at the end of the book.

Schedule I Drugs   Schedule V Drugs
Schedule II Drugs   Class 1 Recall
Schedule III Drugs   Class 2 Recall
Schedule IV Drugs   Class 3 Recall

1. _____ :   Amphetamines, opium, cocaine, methadone, and various opiates are included on this schedule.

2. _____ :   Anabolic steroids and various compounds containing limited quantities of narcotic substances such as codeine are included on this schedule.

3. _____ :   When a product is not likely to cause adverse effects.

4. _____ :   Compounds containing limited amounts of a narcotic such as codeine are included in this group.

5. _____ :   When a product may cause temporary but reversible adverse effects, or in which there is little likelihood of serious adverse effects.

6. _____ :   Heroin, various opium derivatives, and hallucinogenic substances are included on this schedule.

7. _____ :   Phenobarbital, the sedative chloral hydrate, and the anesthetic methohexital are included in this group.

8. _____ :   When there is a strong likelihood that the product will cause serious adverse effects or death.

IDENTIFY

Identify the required elements on this manufacturer's bottle label by answering in the space beneath the question.

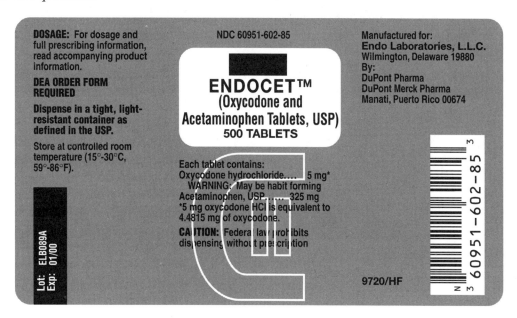

1. In what kind of container should this medication be dispensed?

2. Who is the manufacturer of this drug product?

3. What is the product's brand name?

4. What is the product's generic name?

5. What is the drug form?

6. What are the active ingredients?

7. What control level is the drug product?

8. What are the storage requirements?

9. What is the expiration date?

— 4 —

PHARMACEUTICAL TERMINOLOGY

KEY CONCEPTS

Test your knowledge by covering the information in the right hand column.

terminology	Much of medical science is made up of a small number of root words, suffixes and prefixes that originated from either Greek or Latin words.
root word	The base component of a term which gives it a meaning that may be modified by other components.
prefix	A modifying component of a term located before the other components of the term.
suffix	A modifying component of a term located after the other components of the term.
combining vowel	Combining vowels are used to connect the prefix, root, or suffix parts of the term.
cardiovascular system	Distributes blood throughout the body using blood vessels called arteries, capillaries, and veins.
endocrine system	Consists of the glands that secrete hormones (chemicals that assist in regulating body functions).
gastrointestinal (GI) tract	Contains the organs that are involved in the digestion of foods and the absorption of nutrients.
integumentary system	The body's first line of defense, acting as a barrier against disease and other hazards.
lymphatic system	The center of the body's immune system. Lymphocytes are a white blood cell that helps the body defend itself against bacteria and diseased cells.
muscular system	The body contains more than 600 muscles which give shape and movement to it.

nervous system | The body's system of communication. The neuron (nerve cell) is its basic functional unit.

skeletal system | Protects soft organs and provides structure and support for the body's organ systems.

female reproductive system | Produces hormones (estrogen, progesterone), controls menstruation, and provides for childbearing.

male reproductive system | Produces sperm and secretes the hormone testosterone.

respiratory system | Brings oxygen into the body through inhalation and expels carbon dioxide gas through exhalation.

urinary system | The primary organ is the kidney, which filters the blood for unwanted material and makes urine.

ear | The sense of hearing, as well as the maintenance of body equilibrium, is performed by the ear.

eyes | The eyelids protect the eye and assist in its lubrication. The conjunctiva is the blood-rich membrane between the eye and the eyelid.

drug classifications | A grouping of a number of drugs that have some properties in common. The same steps in interpreting other medical science terminology can be used to interpret drug classification names.

STUDY NOTES

Use this area to write important points you'd like to remember.

ORGAN SYSTEM ROOTS

CARDIOVASCULAR SYSTEM

angi	vessel
aort	aorta
card	heart
oxy	oxygen
pector	chest
phleb	vein
stenosis	narrowing
thromb	clot
vas(cu)	blood vessel
ven	vein

ENDOCRINE SYSTEM

lipid	fat
nephr	kidney
thym	thymus
adrena	adrenal
gluc	sugar
pancreat	pancreas
somat	body

GASTROINTESTINAL SYSTEM

chol	bile
col	colon
duoden	duodenum
enter	intestine
esophag	esophagus
gastr	stomach
hepat	liver
lapar	abdomen
pancreat	pancreas

INTEGUMENTARY SYSTEM

necr	death (cells, body)
derma	skin
cutane	skin
mast	breast
onych	nail

LYMPHATIC SYSTEM

aden	gland
cyt	cell
hemo, hemat	blood
lymph	lymph
splen	spleen

MUSCULAR SYSTEM

my	muscle
fibr	fiber
tendin	tendon

NERVOUS SYSTEM

cerebr	cerebrum
encephal	brain
mening	meninges
myel	spinal cord
neur	nerve

SKELETAL SYSTEM

arthr	joint
calcane	heel bone
carp	wrist
crani	cranium
dactyl	finger or toe
femor	thigh bone
fibul	small, outer lower leg bone
humer	humerus
myel	bone marrow, spinal cord
oste	bone
patell	kneecap
ped, pod	foot
pelv	pelvis
phalang	bones of fingers and toes
rachi	spinal cord, vertebrae
spondy	backbone, vertebrae
stern	sternum, breastbone
tibi	large lower leg bone
vertebr	backbone, vertebrae

ORGAN SYSTEM ROOTS

FEMALE REPRODUCTIVE SYSTEM

gynec	woman
hyster	uterus
lact	milk
mamm	breast
mast	breast
metr	uterus
ovari	ovary
salping	fallopian tube
toc	birth
uter	uterine

MALE REPRODUCTIVE SYSTEM

andr	male
balan	glans penis
orchid, test	testis, testicle
prostat	prostate gland
sperm	sperm
vas	vessel, duct
vesicul	seminal vescles

RESPIRATORY SYSTEM

aer	air
aero	gas
pneum	lung, air
pulmon	lung
pector	chest
nasal	nose
sinus	sinus
laryng	larynx
bronch	bronchus
ox	oxygen
capnia	carbon dioxide

URINARY SYSTEM

cyst	bladder
vesic	bladder
ren	kidney
nephr	kidney
uria	urine, urination

HEARING

ot	ear
cusis	hearing condition
acous	hearing
audi	hearing
salping	eustachian tube
tympan	eardrum
myring	eardrum
cerumin	wax-like, waxy

SIGHT

blephar	eyelid
cor	pupil
dacry, lacrim	tear, tear duct
corne, kerat	cornea
retin	retina
irid, iri	iris
bi, bin	two
opia	vision

STUDY NOTES

Use this area to write important points you'd like to remember.

COMMON PREFIXES

a	without		medi	middle
ambi	both		melan	black
an	without		meso	middle
ante	before		meta	beyond, after, changing
anti	against		micro	small
bi	two or both		mid	middle
brady	slow		mono	one
chlor	green		multi	many
circum	around		neo	new
cirrh	yellow		pan	all
con	with		para	alongside or abnormal
contra	against		peri	around
cyan	blue		polio	gray
dia	across or through		poly	many
dis	separate from or apart		post	after
dys	painful, difficult		pre	before
ec	away or out		pro	before
ecto	outside		pseudo	false
end	within		purpur	purple
epi	upon		quadri	four
erythr	red		re	again or back
eu	good or normal		retro	after
exo	outside		rube	red
heter	different		semi	half
hom	same		sub	below or under
hyper	above or excessive		super	above or excessive
hypo	below or deficient		supra	above or excessive
im	not		sym	with
immun	safe, protected		syn	with
in	not		tachy	fast
infra	below or under		trans	across, through
inter	between		tri	three
intra	within		ultra	beyond or excessive
is	equal		uni	one
leuk	white		xanth	yellow
macro	large		xer	dry

COMMON SUFFIXES

ac	pertaining to		oi	resembling
al	pertaining to		ole	small
algia	pain		oma	tumor
ar	pertaining to		opia	vision
ary	pertaining to		opsia	vision
asthenia	without strength		osis	abnormal condition
cele	pouching or hernia		osmia	smell
cyesis	pregnancy		ous	pertaining to
cynia	pain		paresis	partial paralysis
eal	pertaining to		pathy	disease
ectasis	expansion or dilation		penia	decrease
ectomy	removal		phagia	swallowing
emia	blood condition		phasia	speech
gram	record		philia	attraction for
graph	recording instrument		phobia	fear
graphy	recording process		plasia	formation
ia	condition of		plegia	paralysis, stroke
iasis	condition, formation of		rrhea	discharge
iatry	treatment		sclerosis	narrowing, constriction
ic	pertaining to		scope	examination instrument
icle	small		scopy	examination
ism	condition of		spasm	involuntary contraction
itis	inflammation		stasis	stop or stand
ium	tissue		tic	pertaining to
lith	stone, calculus		tocia	childbirth, labor
logy	study of		tomy	incision
malacia	softening		toxic	poison
megaly	enlargement		tropic	stimulate
meter	measuring instrument		ula	small
metry	measuring process		y	condition, process

COMMON PHARMACY ABBREVIATIONS

Here are the most common abbreviations, with the latin term where there is one.

ROUTE

a.d.	right ear
a.s.	left ear
a.u.	each ear
i.m., IM	intramuscular
inj.	injection
i.v., IV	intravenous
i.v.p., IVP	intravenous push
IVPB	intravenous piggyback
o.d.	right eye
o.s.	left eye
o.u.	each eye
p.o.	by mouth
SC, SQ	subcutaneously
top.	topically, locally

FORM

aq	water
aqua. dist.	distilled water
caps	capsules
DW	distilled water
elix.	elixir
liq.	liquid
NS	normal saline
supp.	suppository
syr.	syrup
tab.	tablet
ung.	ointment

TIME

a.c.	before food, before meals
a.m.	morning
a.t.c.	around the clock
b.i.d.,bid	twice a day
h	hour, at the hour of
h.s.	at bedtime
p.c.	after food, after meals
p.r.n., prn	as needed
q.i.d., qid	four times a day
q	each, every
q.d.	every day
q.h.	every hour
stat.	immediately
t.i.d., tid	three times a day

MEASUREMENT

$\bar{\imath}$	one
a.a. or aa	of each
ad	to, up to
aq. ad	add water up to
dil.	dilute
div.	divide
f, fl.	fluid
g., G., gm.	gram
gtt.	drop
L	liter
mcg.	microgram
mEq.	milliequivalent
mg.	milligram
ml.	milliliter
q.s.	a sufficient quantity
qsad	add sufficient quantity to make
ss	one-half
tbsp.	tablespoon
tsp.	teaspoon

OTHER

c	with
d.t.d.	give of such doses
disp.	dispense
f, ft.	make, let it be made
l	left
s	without
ut dict., u.d.	as directed
sig.	write, label

Note that the use of periods in abbreviations varies greatly. It is important to be able to recognize abbreviations with or without periods.

LESS COMMON PHARMACY ABBREVIATIONS

ad lib.	at pleasure
add	add (thou)
agit	shake, stir
alt. h.	every other hour
a.	before
amp.	ampule
aur.; a	ear
aurist	ear-drops
b.	twice
brach.	the arm
BSA	body surface area
c.c.	cubic centimeter
charts	powder papers; divided powders
cib.; c.	food
collun	a nose wash
collut.	a mouthwash
collyr.	an eyewash
comp.	compound
cong.; C.	gallon
c.c.	with food; with meals
d.	give (thou); let be given
d.	right
dieb. alt.	every other day
emuls.	emulsion
et	and
e.m.p.	in the manner prescribed
gr.	grain
lin.	liniment
lot.	lotion
min;	minum
m.; M	mix
n.	at night
narist.	nasal drops
neb.	a spray
N.F.	National Formulary
non.rep.	do not repeat
O.	pint
occulent.	eye ointment
o.	eye
o.m.	every morning
p.a.a.	to be applied to affected part
p.r.	per rectum
pulv.	powder

s.a.	according to the art
s.o.s.	if necessary
sol.	solution
tinc.; tr.	tincture
troche	lozenge
tuss.	a cough

SOME COMMON MEDICAL ABBREVIATIONS

AIDS	Acquired immunodeficiency syndrome
AV	Atrial-ventricular
AMI	Acute myocardial infarction
ANS	Autonomic nervous system
BM	Bowel movement
BP	Blood pressure
CA	Cancer
COPD	Chronic obstructive pulmonary disease
CV	Cardiovascular
CVA	Cerebrovascular accident (stroke)
DI	Diabetes insipidus
DOB	Date of birth
DX	Diagnosis
ECG, EKG	Electrocardiogram
GERD	Gastroesophageal reflux disease
GI	Gastrointestinal
H	Hypodermic
HDL	High density lipoprotein
HIV	Human Immunodeficiency virus
IH	Infectious hepatitis
IO, I/O	Fluid intake and output
LDL	Low density lipoprotein
MI	Myocardial infarction
NPO	Nothing by mouth
PUD	Peptic ulcer disease
RBC	Red blood count or red blood cell
T	Temperature
TB	Tuberculosis
U	Units
VD	Venereal disease
WBC	White blood count or white blood cell
WT	Weight
XX	Female sex chromosome
XY	Male sex chromosome

FILL IN THE BLANK

Answers are at the end of the book.

a.a. or aa	1. _____		liq.	33. _____
a.c.	2. _____		mcg.	34. _____
a.d.	3. _____		mEq.	35. _____
a.m.	4. _____		mg.	36. _____
a.s.	5. _____		ml.	37. _____
a.t.c.	6. _____		NS	38. _____
a.u.	7. _____		o.d.	39. _____
ad	8. _____		o.s.	40. _____
aq	9. _____		o.u.	41. _____
aq. ad	10. _____		p.c.	42. _____
aqua. dist.	11. _____		p.o.	43. _____
bid	12. _____		prn	44. _____
c	13. _____		q	45. _____
caps	14. _____		q.d.	46. _____
d.t.d.	15. _____		q.h.	47. _____
dil.	16. _____		qid	48. _____
disp.	17. _____		q.s.	49 _____
div.	18. _____		qsad	50. _____
DW	19. _____		s	51. _____
elix.	20. _____		SC, SQ	52. _____
f, fl.	21. _____		ss	53. _____
g., G., gm.	22. _____		stat.	54. _____
gtt.	23. _____		supp.	55. _____
h	24. _____		syr.	56. _____
h.s.	25. _____		tid	57. _____
i.m., IM	26. _____		tab.	58. _____
i.v., IV	27. _____		tbsp.	59. _____
i.v.p., IVP	28. _____		top.	60. _____
inj.	29 _____		tsp.	61. _____
IVPB	30. _____		ung.	62. _____
L.	31. _____		u.d.	63. _____
l.	32. _____			

FILL IN THE KEY TERM

Use these key terms to fill in the correct blank. Answers are at the end of the book.

anorexia	endocrine	hypothyroidism	sinusitis
arteriosclerosis	endometriosis	leukemia	somatic
bronchitis	gastritis	lymphoma	subcutaneous
cardiomyopathy	hematoma	neuralgia	tendinitis
colitis	hemophilia	osteoarthritis	thrombosis
conjunctivitis	hepatitis	phlebitis	transdermal
cystitis	hyperlipidemia	prostatitis	uremia
dermatitis	hypertension	pulmonary	vaginitis

1. _____ : high blood pressure.
2. _____ : condition of having blood clots in the vascular system.
3. _____ : inflammation of a vein.
4. _____ : hardening of the arteries.
5. _____ : disease of the heart muscle.
6. _____ : pertaining to the glands that secrete onto the bloodstream.
7. _____ : abnormally high amounts of fats in the blood.
8. _____ : a deficiency of thyroid secretion.
9. _____ : pertaining to the body.
10. _____ : loss of appetite.
11. _____ : inflamed or irritable colon.
12. _____ : inflammation of the liver from various causes.
13. _____ : inflammation of the stomach.
14. _____ : skin inflammation.
15. _____ : beneath the skin.
16. _____ : through the skin.
17. _____ : a collection of blood, often clotted.
18. _____ : a disease in which the blood does not clot normally.
19. _____ : lymphatic system tumor.
20. _____ : a disease of blood forming tissues.
21. _____ : inflammation of a tendon.
22. _____ : severe pain in a nerve.
23. _____ : chronic disease of bones and joints.
24. _____ : abnormal growth of uteral tissue within the pelvis.
25. _____ : inflammation of the vagina.
26. _____ : inflammation of prostate.
27. _____ : inflammation of bronchial membranes.
28. _____ : pertaining to the lungs.
29. _____ : inflammation of the sinuses.
30. _____ : inflammation of the bladder.
31. _____ : toxic blood condition caused by kidney disorders.
32. _____ : inflammation of the conjunctiva.

— 5 —

PRESCRIPTIONS

KEY CONCEPTS

Test your knowledge by covering the information in the right hand column.

prescription	A written order from a practitioner for the preparation and administration of a medicine or a device. Medical doctors (MD), dentists (DDS), veterinarians (DVM), and doctors of osteopathy (DO) are the primary practitioners allowed to write prescriptions. In some states, nurse practitioners, physicians assistants, and/or pharmacists are also allowed limited rights to prescribe medications.
medication orders	Used in institutional settings instead of a prescription form.
technician responsibilities	In community pharmacies, this generally includes receiving the prescription, collecting patient data, entering it into a computerized prescription system, and filling orders.
pharmacist role	Does all consulting with patients, handles Schedule II prescriptions, and checks all filled orders before dispensing.
prescription verification	It is necessary to check with the pharmacist on potential forgeries, on prescriptions that are more than a few days old, or on prescriptions that in any way appear questionable.
online billing	A prescription is interpreted and confirmed by the prescription system. If third party billing is involved, this is done online simultaneously.
preparation	Once the prescription and third-party billing is confirmed, the label and receipt are printed and the prescription is prepared.
label	The general purpose of the prescription label is to provide information to the patient regarding the dispensed medication and how to take it. Additionally, the label includes information about the pharmacy, the patient, the prescriber, and the prescription or transaction number assigned to the prescription.

signa	Directions for use. Since the patient is expected to self-administer the medication, these must be clear and easily understood by the patient.
pharmacist check	If a prescription has been prepared by a technician, there is a final check by the pharmacist to make sure that it is correct.
institutional settings	There are different requirements for institutional prescriptions since nursing staff generally administer medications to patients. Rules for institutional pharmacy prescription labels vary by institution but often do not contain much more than the name, strength, manufacturer, expiration date, and dosage form of the medication.
OTC prescriptions	Prescriptions may be written for over-the-counter (OTC) medications.
judgment questions	Technicians must request the advice of the pharmacist whenever judgment is required.
labels	Computer-generated prescription labels must be placed on containers so they are easy to locate and easy to read.
auxiliary labels	Many computerized prescription systems will automatically indicate which auxiliary labels to use with each drug.
controlled substance labels	Schedules II, III and IV substances must carry an auxiliary label stating: "Caution: Federal law prohibits the transfer of this drug to any person other than the patient for whom it was prescribed."

STUDY NOTES

Use this area to write important points you'd like to remember.

THE PRESCRIPTION

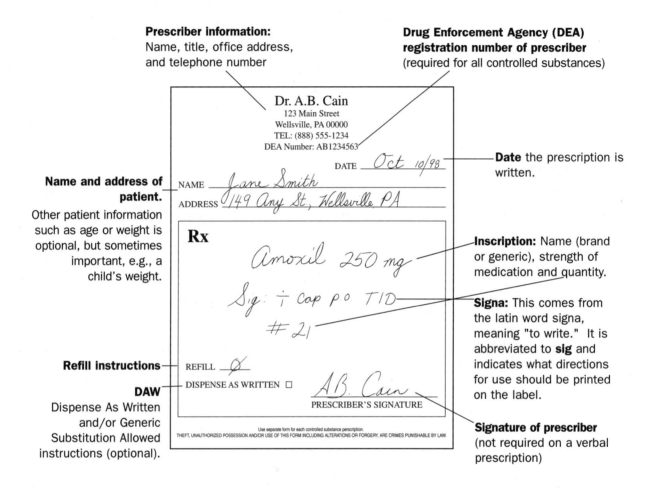

Prescriber information:
Name, title, office address, and telephone number

Drug Enforcement Agency (DEA) registration number of prescriber (required for all controlled substances)

Date the prescription is written.

Name and address of patient.
Other patient information such as age or weight is optional, but sometimes important, e.g., a child's weight.

Inscription: Name (brand or generic), strength of medication and quantity.

Signa: This comes from the latin word signa, meaning "to write." It is abbreviated to **sig** and indicates what directions for use should be printed on the label.

Refill instructions

DAW
Dispense As Written and/or Generic Substitution Allowed instructions (optional).

Signature of prescriber (not required on a verbal prescription)

Note: If a compound is prescribed, a list of ingredients and directions for mixing is included.

Note: prescriptions are written in ink, never pencil.

PRESCRIPTION LABELS

the name, address, and telephone number of the pharmacy

the date dispensed

DEA number

a prescription and/or transaction number

the name of the patient for whom the medication is dispensed

directions for use that are clear and accurate

the name, quantity, strength, manufacturer (name or NDC number), and dosage form of the medication dispensed

expiration date of the medication

the name of the prescriber

refill information.

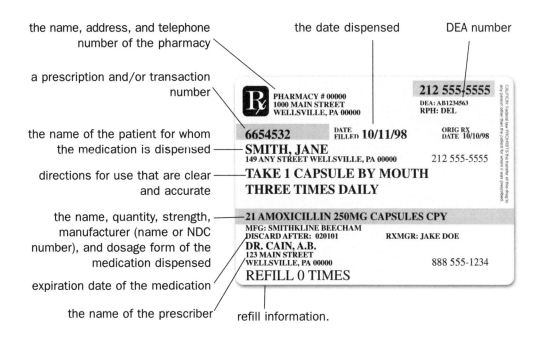

AUXILIARY LABELS

Additional, often colored auxiliary labels may also be applied to the prescription container in order to provide additional information to the patient (e.g. Shake Well, Keep Refrigerated, Take With Food or Milk). Many computerized prescription systems will automatically indicate which auxiliary labels to use.

Controlled substances from schedules II, III and IV must carry an auxiliary label stating:

Caution: Federal law prohibits the transfer of this drug to any person other than the patient for whom it was prescribed.

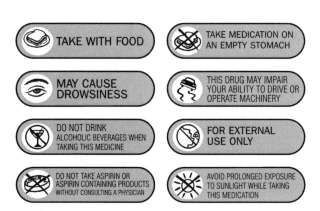

FILL IN THE KEY TERM

Use these key terms to fill in the correct blank. Answers are at the end of the book.

auxiliary label	institutional labels	protocols
DAW	lookalikes	Rx
DEA number	medication orders	Schedules II, III and IV auxiliary
extemporaneous compounding	prescription	label statement
inscription	prescription number	signa

1. _____ : A written order from a practitioner for the preparation and administration of a medicine or a device

2. _____ : The pharmaceutical preparation of a medication from ingredients.

3. _____ : Specific guidelines for practice

4. _____ : The directions for use on a prescription that should be printed on the label.

5. _____ : The additional warning labels that are placed on filled prescription containers.

6. _____ : The form used to prescribe medications for patients in institutional settings.

7. _____ : Drug names that have similar appearance, particularly when written.

8. _____ : Name (brand or generic), strength of medication and quantity.

9. _____ : Dispense As Written, meaning generic substitution not allowed.

10. _____ : An abbreviation of the latin word recipe, meaning "take."

11. _____ : Often do not contain much more than the name, strength, manufacturer, expiration date, and dosage form of the medication.

12. _____ : Caution: Federal law prohibits the transfer of this drug to any person other than the patient for whom it was prescribed.

13. _____ : The number assigned to each prescription which appears on the label.

14. _____ : Required on all controlled substance prescriptions.

TRUE/FALSE

Indicate whether the statement is true or false in the blank. Answers are at the end of the book.

_____ 1. In addition to the primary prescribers, nurse practitioners and physician assistants are allowed to write prescriptions in some states.

_____ 2. All prescriptions must be signed by the prescriber.

_____ 3. The signa indicates the medication and its strength.

_____ 4. If DAW is indicated, generic substitution may not be used.

_____ 5. A prescription has no time limit.

_____ 6. Patients with OTC prescriptions should be referred to the pharmacist.

_____ 7. One of the primary purposes of the prescription label is to provide the patient with clear instructions on how to take the medication.

_____ 8. Institutional labels must have the same information as in the community setting.

_____ 9. The prescription label may have either the date dispensed or the expiration date, but does not need both.

_____ 10. A DEA number is required on all prescriptions.

EXPLAIN WHY

Explain why these statements are true or important. Check your answers in the text. Discuss any questions you may have with your Instructor.

1. Why must the pharmacist always check the filled prescription before it is dispensed to the patient?

2. Why must the directions for use be clear and understandable to the patient in the community setting?

3. What are the differences between the prescription and the medication order? Why?

4. Why must prescriptions be written in ink?

5. Why are auxiliary labels important?

IDENTIFY

Identify the elements on this medication order by answering in the space beneath the question.

		PATIENT IDENTIFICATION	
DOCTOR'S ORDERS		099999999 675-01 SMITH, JOHN 12/06/1950 DR. P. JOHNSON	

DATE	TIME	DOCTOR'S ORDERS ①	DATE/TIME INITIALS	DATE/TIME INITIALS
1/5/99	22⁰⁰	Admit patient to 6ᵗʰ floor		
		Pneumonia, Dehydration		
		All: PCN - Rash		
		Order CBC, chem-7, blood cultures stat		
		Start D5-NS @ 125 ml/hr IV q8°		
		Dr Johnson X2222		

DATE	TIME	DOCTOR'S ORDERS ②	DATE/TIME INITIALS	DATE/TIME INITIALS
2/6/99	3⁰⁰	Tylenol 650mg po q4-6 hrs PRN for Temp > 38°C		
		Verbal Order Dr Johnson/ Jane Doe, RN		

DATE	TIME	DOCTOR'S ORDERS ③	DATE/TIME INITIALS	DATE/TIME INITIALS
2/6/99	6⁰⁰	Start Clarithromycin 500mg po q12°		
		Multivitamin po qd		
		Order CXR for this a.m.		
		Dr Johnson X2222		

1. What is the patient's disorder/condition?

2. Does the patient have allergies?

3. What route and dosage is ordered for the Tylenol 650mg?

4. What orders did the physician sign for?

5. What route and dosage are prescribed for the Clarithromycin?

6. What route and dosage are prescribed for the multivitamin?

7. What is the time span of these orders?

IDENTIFY

Identify the elements on this prescription by answering in the space beneath the question.

Dr. A.B. Cain
123 Main Street
Wellsville, PA 00000
TEL: (888) 555-1234
DEA Number: AB1234563

DATE *Oct 6/98*

NAME *Scott Barr*

ADDRESS *345 Maple St, Wellsville PA*
D.O.B – 2/23/54

Rx

Prozac 20 mg

Sig: ī cap p.o. qd

 # 30

REFILL *X2*

DISPENSE AS WRITTEN ☑   *A.B. Cain*

PRESCRIBER'S SIGNATURE

Use separate form for each controlled substance perscription.
THEFT, UNAUTHORIZED POSSESSION AND/OR USE OF THIS FORM INCLUDING ALTERATIONS OR FORGERY, ARE CRIMES PUNISHABLE BY LAW.

1. What is the name of the drug?

2. What is the strength?

3. What is the dosage form?

4. What is the route of administration?

5. What is the dosage?

6. How many refills are there?

7. Can there be generic substitution?

— 6 —

Calculations

RATIO AND PROPORTION

Most of the calculations pharmacy technicians will face on the job or in the certification exam can be performed using the *ratio and proportion* method.

A ratio states a relationship between two quantities. ➡ $\dfrac{a}{b}$

A proportion contains two equal ratios. ➡ $\dfrac{a}{b} = \dfrac{c}{d}$

When three of the four quantities in a proportion are known, the value of the fourth (x) can be easily solved. ➡ $\dfrac{x}{b} = \dfrac{c}{d}$

CONDITIONS FOR USING RATIO AND PROPORTION

1. Three of the four values must be known.

2. Numerators must have the same units.

3. Denominators must have the same units.

STEPS FOR SOLVING PROPORTION PROBLEMS

1. Define the variable and correct ratios.

2. Set-up the proportion equation

3. Establish the x equation

4. Solve for x.

5. Express solution in correct units.

Example

If there are 125 mg of a substance in a 500 ml solution, and 50 mg is desired, the amount of solution needed can be determined with this equation:

$$\frac{x \text{ ml}}{50 \text{ mg}} = \frac{500 \text{ ml}}{125 \text{ mg}}$$

multiplying both sides by 50 mg gives:

x ml = 2500 ml/125

solving for x gives:

x = 200

answer: 200 ml of solution are needed.

CONVERSIONS

Many proportion problems involve the use of conversions from one unit of measure to another. Here is a list of the most common.

Liquid Metric

1L	=	10dl	=	1000ml
1dl	=	.1L	=	100ml
1ml	=	.001L	=	.01dl

Solid Metric

1 kg	=	1,000 g		
1 g	=	.001 kg	=	1,000 mg
1 mg	=	.001 g	=	1,000 mcg
1 mcg	=	.001 mg		

Avoirdupois

1 lb	=	16 oz
1 oz	=	437.5 gr
1 gr	=	64.8 mg (.0648 g)

Apothecary

1 gal	=	4 qt
1 qt	=	2 pt
1 pt	=	16 fl oz
1 fl oz	=	8 fl dr
1 fl dr	=	60 m

Household

1 tsp	=	5ml		
1 tbs	=	3 tsp	=	15ml
1 cup	=	8 fl oz		

Temperature

F temperature $= (1\frac{4}{5}$ times number of degrees C) + 32

C temperature $= \frac{5}{9}$ x (number of degrees F - 32)

Conversions Between Systems

1 L	=	33.8 fl oz		1 lb	=	453.59 g
1 pt	=	473.167 ml		1 oz	=	28.35 g
1 fl oz	=	29.57ml		1 g	=	15.43 gr
1 kg	=	2.2 lb		1 gr	=	64.8 mg

ROMAN NUMERALS

Roman numerals can be capital or lower case letters, and are:

ss = 1/2	L or l = 50
I or i = 1	C or c = 100
V or v = 5	D or d = 500
X or x = 10	M or m = 1000

RULES:

➡ When the second of two letters has a value equal to or smaller than that of the first, their values are to be added.

➡ When the second of two letters has a value greater than that of the first, the smaller is to be subtracted from the larger.

CONVERSION EXERCISES

Convert these numbers to decimals:

1. 1 1/4 _____
2. 0.5% _____
3. 6/8 _____
4. 2/3 _____
5. 8% _____
6. 42.5% _____
7. 3.2% _____

Write the following in Roman numerals:

15. 4 _____
16. 49 _____
17. 62 _____
18. 108 _____
19. 24 _____
20. 98 _____
21. 14 _____

Convert these numbers to percents:

8. .008 _____
9. 3/6 _____
10. 0.042 _____
11. 1/8 _____
12. 0.075 _____
13. 2/5 _____
14. 0.025 _____

Write the following in arabic numbers:

22. XXIV _____
23. CIV _____
24. MCC _____
25. iiss _____
26. XVIII _____
27. LIV _____

PROBLEMS

1. You have a prescription that calls for 1 cap po qid x 10 days. How many capsules are needed?

2. You have a prescription that calls for 1 cap po tid x 7 days. How many capsules are needed?

3. If a compounding order calls for Flagyl® 125 mg bid x 7 days, and only 0.5 gm tablets are available, how many tablets will it take to fill the order?

4. How much talc is needed for an order for 120 gm of the following compound: nupercainal ointment 4%, zinc oxide 20%, talc 2%?

5. A prescription calls for 200 mg of a drug that you have in a 10 mg/15 ml concentration. How many ml of the liquid do you need?

PEDIATRIC DOSES

Because of the many variables, conversion formulas for pediatric doses are rarely used in the pharmacy. Doses are generally given by the physician. **Children's doses are stated by kg of body weight (dose/kg).** Since 1 kg = 2.2 lb, you can solve for the prescribed dose by using a proportion equation if you know the child's body weight. See the following example.

An antibiotic IV is prescribed for an infant. The dose is to be 15 mg/kg twice a day. The baby weighs 12 lbs. How much drug is to be given for one dose? First the infant's weight in kilograms should be calculated.

$$x \text{ kg} / 12 \text{ lb} = 1 \text{ kg} / 2.2 \text{ lb}$$

$$x \text{ kg} = 12 \text{ lb times } \frac{1 \text{ kg}}{2.2 \text{ lb}} = \frac{12 \text{ kg}}{2.2} = 5.45 \text{ kg}$$

The next part of this problem can be solved with a simple equation.

one dose $= 15 \text{ mg times } 5.45 = 81.75 \text{ mg}$

PERCENTS & SOLUTIONS

Percents are used to indicate the amount or **concentration** of something in a solution. Concentrations are indicated in terms of weight to volume or volume to volume. The standard units are:

Weight to Volume: grams per 100 milliliters ➡ **g/ml**

Volume to Volume: milliliters per 100 milliliters ➡ **ml/ml**

A PERCENT SOLUTION FORMULA

Technicians find that they often have to convert a solution at one concentration to a solution having a different concentration, especially during the preparation of **hyperalimentation** or **TPNs**. It is possible to make such conversions using a simple proportion equation with these elements:

$$\frac{x \text{ volume wanted}}{\text{want \%}} = \frac{\text{volume prescribed}}{\text{have \%}}$$

FLOW RATE

In some settings, the flow rate or rate of administration for an IV solution needs to be calculated. This is done using a ratio and proportion equation. Rates are generally calculated in ml/hour, but for pumps used to dispense IV fluids to a patient, the calculation may need to be done in ml/min or gtt/min.

For example, if you have an order for KCl 10 mEq and K Acetate 15 mEq in D5W 1000 ml to run at 80 ml/hour, you would determine the administration rate in ml/minute as follows:

x ml / 1 min = 80 ml / 60 min

x = 80/60 = 1.33

To get **drops per minute (gtt/min)**, you must have a conversion rate of drops per ml. For example, if the administration set for the above order delivered 30 drops per ml, you would find the drops per minute as follows:

$$\frac{80 \text{ ml}}{60 \text{ min}} \times \frac{30 \text{ gtt}}{1 \text{ ml}} = \frac{2400 \text{ gtt}}{60 \text{ min}} = 40 \text{ gtt/min}$$

MILLIEQUIVALENT—mEq

Electrolytes are substances which conduct an electrical current and are found in the body's blood, tissue fluids, and cells. Salts are electrolytes and saline solutions are a commonly used electrolyte solution. The concentration of electrolytes in a volume of solution is measured in units called milliequivalents (mEq). They are expressed as milliequivalents per milliliter or equivalents per liter.

Milliequivalents are a unit of measurement specific to each electrolyte. For example, a 0.9% solution of one electrolyte will have a different mEq value than a 0.9% solution of another because mEq values are based on each electrolyte's atomic weight and electron properties, each of which is different.

If the mEq value of a solution is known, it is relatively easy to mix it with other solutions to get a different mEq volume ratio by using proportions.

EXAMPLE

A solution calls for 5 mEq of an electrolyte that you have in a 1.04 mEq / ml solution. How many ml of it do you need?

x ml/ 5 mEq = 1 ml/1.04 mEq

x ml = 5 mEq times $\frac{1 \text{ ml}}{1.04 \text{ mEq}}$ = $\frac{5 \text{ ml}}{1.04}$ = 4.8 ml

Answer: 4.8 ml of the solution is needed.

PROBLEMS

Use the preceding information to solve these problems

6. An IV requires the addition of 45 mEq potassium chloride (KCL). You have a vial of KCl at a concentration of 20 mEq per 10 ml. How many mls should be added?

7. If 360 grams of dextrose is ordered using a 50% dextrose solution, how many ml are needed?

8. A prescription calls for 0.36 mg of a drug that you have in 50 mcg/ml concentration. How many ml do you need?

9. The infusion rate of an IV is 300 ml over 4 hours. What is the ml/minute rate?

10. The infusion rate of an IV is 1000 ml over 12 hours. What is the rate per minute?

11. An IV order calls for administration of 1.5 ml/minute of a solution for four hours. How much solution will be needed.

12. If a physician orders 35% dextrose 1000 ml and all you have is 70% dextrose 1000 ml, how much 70% dextrose and how much sterile water will be used?

13. If a physician orders 20% dextrose 1000 ml and all you have is 70% dextrose 1000 ml, how much 70% dextrose and how much sterile water will be used?

14. If a physician orders 25% Dextrose 500 ml and you have 50% Dextrose 1000ml, how much 50% Dextrose and how much sterile water do you need?

TOTAL PARENTERAL NUTRITION

A TPN order calls for the amounts on the left (including additives) to be made from the items on the right. The total volume is to be 1000 ml. How much of each ingredient and how much sterile water do you need to prepare this TPN ?

TPN Order	On Hand	
aminosyn 4.25%	aminosyn 8.5%	1000 ml
dextrose 20%	dextrose 50%	500 ml

Additives:

KCl	24 mEq	KCl 2mEq/ml	20 ml
MVI	5 ml	MVI	10 ml
NaCl	24 mEq	NaCl 4.4mEq/ml	20 ml

Figure out the amounts and enter the answer on the blank line.

1.) aminosyn _____

2.) dextrose _____

3.) KCl _____

4.) MVI _____

5.) NaCl _____

6.) sterile water _____

EXAMINATION NOTE: ALLIGATIONS

One type of problem that may appear on the certification exam specifies the use of the **alligation method** for mixing solutions of different concentrations. For example, how much of a 95% solution should be mixed with a 50% solution to create a 70% solution? Here's how to solve this using the alligation method.

a) Determine "**y**" (the amount needed of the weaker solution) by subtracting the desired solution concentration from the concentration with the highest percentage:
95-70 = 25

b) Determine "**x**" (the amount needed of the stronger solution) by subtracting the weaker solution concentration from the desired solution concentration:
70-50 = 20

c) The **x/y ratio is therefore 20/25**, with x indicating the number of parts of the higher percentage solution and y indicating the number of parts of the lower pecentage solution needed for the mixture.

d) Intepret this as **20 parts of the 95% solution are needed for every 25 of the 50% solution.** (This can also be reduced to four parts of one for every five of the other.)

RETAIL MATH

Technicians in community pharmacies must know how to perform common retail calculations. Besides simple addition and subtraction, the most important calculations involve using percentages, especially in doing **mark-ups** or **discounts**. A mark-up is the amount of the retailer's selling price minus their purchase price. It is calculated by multiplying the retailer's purchase price by the mark-up percentage and adding the amount to the cost.

For example, a 30% mark-up on an item purchased for $2.30 is $0.69 (Note that 30% equals 0.3, and that $2.30 x 0.3 = $0.69), so the selling price would be $2.99 ($2.30 + $0.69).

Conversely, if you knew a $2.99 sale item was marked-up $0.69 and were asked to figure out the percent mark-up, you would subtract the $0.69 from $2.99 to get the cost of the item ($2.30), and then divide the mark-up by the cost: $0.69 ÷ $2.30 = 0.3 = 30%.

Discounts involve subtracting a percentage amount from the marked-up price of an item. A 30% discount on the $2.99 item is $0.90, so $2.09 would be the discounted price ($2.99-$0.90). Note that this is different than the cost of the item, because you deducted the percentage from the marked-up price.

—7—

ROUTES AND FORMULATIONS

KEY CONCEPTS

Test your knowledge by covering the information in the right hand column.

formulations	Drugs are contained in products called formulations. There are many drug formulations and many different routes to administer them.
route of administration	Routes are classified as enteral or parenteral. Enteral refers to anything involving the tract from the mouth to the rectum. There are three enteral routes: oral, sublingual, and rectal. Any route other than oral, sublingual, and rectal is considered a parenteral administration route. Oral administration is the most frequently used route of administration.
local and systemic effects	A local effect occurs when the drug activity is at the site of administration (e.g., eyes, ears, nose, skin). A systemic effect occurs when the drug is introduced into the circulatory system.
oral administration	The stomach has a pH around 1-2. Certain drugs cannot be taken orally because they are degraded or destroyed by stomach acid and intestinal enzymes. Drugs administered by liquid dosage forms generally reach the circulatory system faster than drugs formulated in solid dosage forms.
oral formulations	Oral formulations contain various ingredients beside the active drug. These inactive ingredients include binders, effervescent salts, lubricants, fillers, diluents, and disintegrants.
gastrointestinal action	The disintegration and dissolution of tablets, capsules, and powders generally begins in the stomach, but will continue to occur when the stomach empties into the intestine. Controlled-release or extended-release formulations extend dissolution over a period of hours and provide a longer duration of effect compared to plain tablets. Enteric coated tablets prevent the tablet from disintegrating until it reaches the higher pHs of the intestine.

sublingual administration

These tablets are placed under the tongue. They are generally fast dissolving uncoated tablets which contain highly water soluble drugs. When the drug is released from the tablet, it is quickly absorbed into the circulatory system since the membranes lining the mouth are very thin and there is a rich blood supply to the mouth.

rectal administration

Rectal administration may be used to achieve a variety of systemic effects, including: asthma control, antinausea, anti-motion sickness, and anti-infective. However, absorption from rectal administration is erratic and unpredictable. The most common rectal administration forms are suppositories, solutions, and ointments.

parenteral administration

Parenteral routes are often preferred when oral administration causes drug degradation or when a rapid drug response is desired, as in an emergency situation. The parenteral routes requiring a needle are intravenous, intramuscular, intradermal, and subcutaneous. These solutions must be sterile (bacteria-free), have an appropriate pH, and be limited in volume.

intravenous formulations

Intravenous dosage forms are administered directly into a vein (and the blood supply). Most solutions are aqueous (water based), but they may also have glycols, alcohols, or other non-aqueous solvents in them.

IV emulsions

Fat emulsions and TPN emulsions are used to provide triglycerides, fatty acids, and calories for patients who cannot absorb them from the gastrointestinal tract.

infusion

Infusion is the gradual intravenous injection of a volume of fluid into a patient.

intravenous sites

Several sites on the body are used to intravenously administer drugs: the veins of the antecubital area (in front of the elbow), the back of the hand, and some of the larger veins in the foot. On some occasions, a vein must be exposed by a surgical cut.

intramuscular injections

The principal sites of injection are the gluteal (buttocks), deltoid (upper arm), and vastus lateralis (thigh) muscles. Intramuscular injections generally result in lower but longer lasting blood concentrations than after intravenous administration.

subcutaneous injections

Injection sites include the back of the upper arm, the front of the thigh, the lower portion of the abdomen and the upper back. The subcutaneous (SC, SQ) route can be used for both short term and very long term therapies. Insulin is the most important drug routinely administered by this route.

Test your knowledge by covering the information in the right hand column.

intradermal injections

Intradermal injections involve small volumes that are injected into the top layer of skin. The usual site for intradermal injections is the rear of the forearm.

ophthalmic formulations

Every ophthalmic product must be manufactured to be sterile in its final container. A major problem of ophthalmic administration is the immediate loss of a dose by natural spillage from the eye.

intranasal formulations

Intranasal formulations are primarily used for their decongestant activity on the nasal mucosa, the cellular lining of the nose. The drugs that are typically used are decongestants, antihistamines, and corticosteroids. Since nasal administration often causes amounts of the drug to be swallowed, in some cases this may lead to a systemic effect.

inhalations formulations

Inhalation dosage forms are intended to deliver drugs to the pulmonary system (lungs). Most of the inhalation dosage forms are aerosols that depend on the power of compressed or liquefied gas to expel the drug from the container. Gaseous or volatile anesthetics are the most important drugs administered via this route. Other drugs administered affect lung function, act as bronchodilators (bronchial tube decongestants), or treat allergic symptoms. Examples of drugs administered by this route are adrenocorticoid steroids (beclomethasone), bronchodilators (epinephrine, isoproterenol, metaproterenol, albuterol), and antiallergics (cromolyn).

dermal formulations

Most dermal dosage forms are used for local (topical) effects on or within the skin. Dermal formulations are used to treat minor skin infections, itching, burns, diaper rash, insect stings and bites, athlete's foot, corns, calluses, warts, dandruff, acne, psoriasis, and eczema. The major disadvantage of this route of administration is that the amount of drug that can be absorbed will be limited to about 2 mg/day.

vaginal administration

Formulations for this route of administration are: solutions, powders for solutions, ointments, creams, aerosol foams, suppositories, tablets, contraceptive sponges and IUDs. Vaginal administration leads to variable absorption since the vagina is a physiologically and anatomically dynamic organ with pH and absorption characteristics changing over time. Another disadvantage of this route is that administration of a formulation during menstruation could predispose the patient to Toxic Shock Syndrome.

TRUE/FALSE

Indicate whether the statement is true or false in the blank. Answers are at the end of the book.

_____ 1. Sublingual administration is a parenteral route of administration.

_____ 2. Oral administration is the most frequently used route of administration.

_____ 3. With oral formulations, drugs administered by solid dosage forms generally reach the systemic circulation faster than liquid dosage forms.

_____ 4. A low pH value such as 1 or 2 indicates a high acidity.

_____ 5. Parenteral administration always involves the use of a needle.

_____ 6. Emulsions are used in intravenous administration to deliver triglycerides, fatty acids and calories.

_____ 7. Intramuscular injections generally cause more pain than intravenous injections.

_____ 8. Insulin is routinely administered by the subcutaneous route.

_____ 9. An advantage of ophthalmic administration is that most of the dose is always delivered to the eye.

_____ 10. Nasal formulations only have a local effect on the nasal mucosa.

EXPLAIN WHY

Explain why these statements are true or important. Check your answers in the text. Discuss any questions you may have with your Instructor.

1. Give three reasons why a drug might not be used for oral administration.

2. Give three reasons why a drug might not be used for parenteral administration.

3. Why do most parenterals require skilled personnel to administer them?

4. Why is the pH of intravenous solutions important?

5. Why is the development of infusion pumps important?

6. Why is it difficult to deliver drugs by inhalation?

FILL IN THE KEY TERM

Answers are at the end of the book.

adsorb	intramuscular injection sites	solvent
aqueous	intravenous sites	sterile
biocompatibility	IUD	subcutaneous injection sites
colloids	lacrimal canalicula	sublingual administration
conjunctiva	lacrimal gland	systemic effect
contraceptive	local effect	topical
degradation	metered dose inhalers	Toxic Shock Syndrome
emulsions	nasal cavity	transcorneal transport
enteric coated	nasal inhaler	transdermal patches
hemorrhoid	nasal mucosa	trauma
hydrates	necrosis	viscosity
inactive ingredients	parenteral	water soluble
inspiration	percutaneous	wheal
intradermal injections	pH	

1. _____ : When the drug activity is at the site of administration (e.g., eyes, ears, nose, skin).

2. _____ : When a drug is introduced into the circulatory system by any route of administration and carried to the site of activity.

3. _____ : The changing of a drug to a less effective or ineffective form.

4. _____ : The attachment of one chemical to another.

5. _____ : The scale that measures the acidity or the opposite (alkalinity) of a substance.

6. _____ : Ingredients beside the active drug that include binders, effervescent salts, lubricants, fillers, diluents, and disintegrants.

7. _____ : Coating that will not let the tablet disintegrate until it reaches the higher pHs of the intestine.

8. _____ : The property of a substance being able to dissolve in water.

9. _____ : When tablets are placed under the tongue

10. _____ : Painful swollen veins in the anal/rectal area.

11. _____ : Any route other than oral, sublingual, and rectal.

12. _____ : The death of cells.

13. _____ : Absence of all microorganisms, both harmful and harmless.

14. _____ : Injections administered into the top layer of the skin at a slight angle using short needles.

15. _____ : The veins of the antecubital area (in front of the elbow), the back of the hand, and some of the larger veins in the foot.

16. _____ : Water based.

17. _____ : A liquid that dissolves another substance in it.

18. _____ : An injury.

19. _____ : Particles up to a hundred times smaller than that those in suspensions that are, however, likewise suspended in a solution.

20. _____ : A mixture of two liquids that do not dissolve into each other in which one liquid is spread through the other by mixing and use of a stabilizer.

21. _____ : Gluteal (buttocks), deltoid (upper arm), and vastus lateralis (thigh) muscles.

22. _____ : The back of the upper arm, the front of the thigh, the lower portion of the abdomen and the upper back.

23. _____ : The thickness of a liquid.

24. _____ : Not irritating or infection or abscess causing to body tissue.

25. _____ : A raised blister-like area on the skin, as caused by an intradermal injection.

26. _____ : The gland that produces tears for the eye.

27. _____ : The tear ducts.

28. _____ : The eyelid lining.

29. _____ : Drug transfer into the eye.

30. _____ : The cellular lining of the nose.

31. _____ : The space behind the nose and above the roof of the mouth that filters air and moves mucous and inhaled contaminants outward and away from the lungs.

32. _____ : A device which contains a drug that is vaporized by inhalation.

33. _____ : Breathing in.

34. _____ : Aerosols that use special metering valves to deliver a fixed dose when the aerosol is activated.

35. _____ : The absorption of drugs through the skin, often for a systemic effect.

36. _____ : Applied for local effect, usually to the skin.

37. _____ : Absorbs water.

38. _____ : Deliver drugs through the skin for a systemic effect.

39. _____ : A rare and potentially fatal disease that results from a severe bacterial infection of the blood.

40. _____ : A device or formulation designed to prevent pregnancy.

41. _____ : An intrauterine contraceptive device that is placed in the uterus for a prolonged period of time.

IDENTIFY

Identify the route of administration.

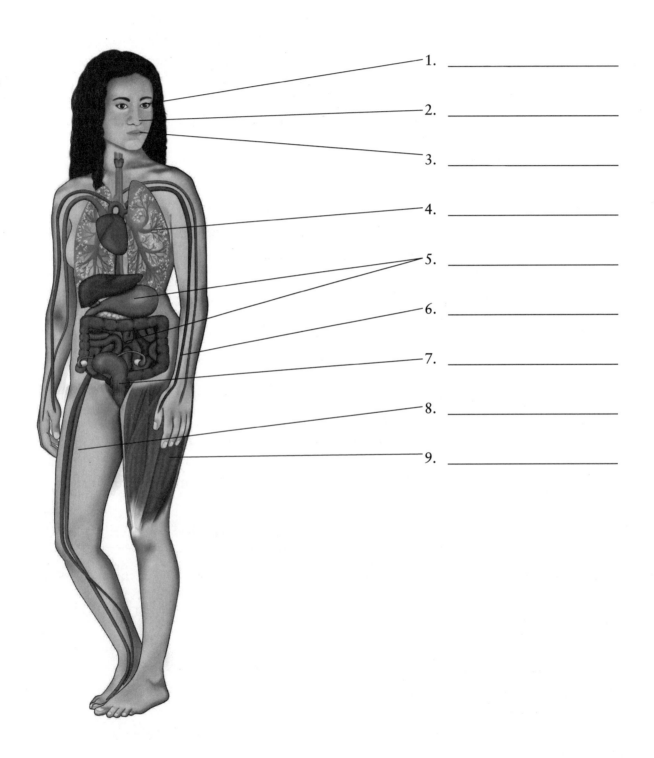

1. _____

2. _____

3. _____

4. _____

5. _____

6. _____

7. _____

8. _____

9. _____

IDENTIFY

Identify the routes of administration.

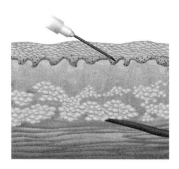

1. _____

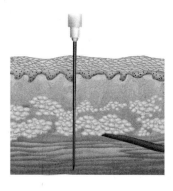

4. _____

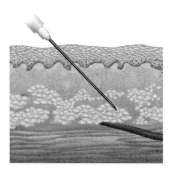

2. _____

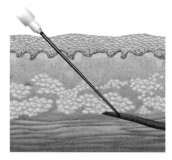

3. _____

Identify these sites of intramuscular administration on the figure at right:

1. deltoid _____

2. gluteus maximus _____

3. gluteus medius _____

4. vastus lateralis _____

5. ventrogluteal _____

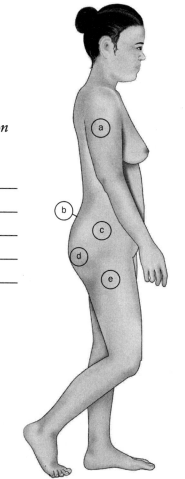

— 8 —

PARENTERALS

KEY CONCEPTS

Test your knowledge by covering the information in the right hand column.

parenteral solutions	There are two types of products: large volume parenteral (LVP) solutions and small volume parenteral (SVP) solutions. LVP solutions are typically bags or bottles containing larger volumes of intravenous solutions. SVP solutions are generally contained in ampules or vials.
properties	Solutions for injection or infusion must be sterile, free of visible particulate material, pyrogen-free, stable for their intended use, have a pH around 7.4, and in most (but not all) cases isotonic.
flow rate	The rate at which the solution is administered to the patient.
piggybacks	Small volumes of fluid (usually 50-100 ml) infused into the administration set of an LVP solution.
pumps	Infusion pumps, syringe pumps, and ambulatory pumps are devices used to administer LVP solutions and control flow rates. Administration sets are threaded through infusion pumps, and the pumps control the gravity flow. Infusion pumps have made the infusion process much more accurate and easier to administer and have been a major factor in the growth of home infusion.
admixtures	When a drug is added to a parenteral solution, the drug is referred to as the additive, and the final mixture is referred to as the admixture.
syringes	Syringes come in sizes ranging from 1 to 60 ml. As a rule, a syringe size is used that is one size larger than the volume to be measured. The volume of solution in a syringe is measured to the edge of the plunger's stopper while the syringe is held upright and all air has been removed from the syringe.
needle sizes	Needle sizes are indicated by length and gauge. The higher the gauge number, the smaller is the lumen (the hollow bore of the needle shaft). Large needles may be needed with highly viscous solutions but are more likely to cause coring.

filters	Often used to remove contaminating particles from solutions. Depth filters and membrane filters are the two basic groups.
laminar flow hood	Establishes and maintains an ultraclean work area for the preparation of IV admixtures.
aseptic techniques	Maintain the sterility of all sterile items and are used in preparing IV admixtures.
biological safety hoods	Used in the preparation of hazardous drugs. They protect both personnel and the environment from contamination.
percentage concentrations	Refer to the drug's weight per 100 ml if the drug is a solid, or the drug's volume per 100 ml if the drug is a liquid.
electrolyte solutions	Equivalent (Eq) or milliequivalent (mEq/l) are used to describe concentrations of electrolytes in solution.
parenteral nutrition solutions	These are complex admixtures composed of dextrose, fat, protein, electrolytes, vitamins, and trace elements. They are hypertonic solutions. Most of the volume of TPN solutions is made up of macronutrients: amino acid solution (a source of protein) and a dextrose solution (a source of carbohydrate calories). Several electrolytes, trace elements, and multiple vitamins (together referred to as micronutrients) may be added to the base solution to meet individual patient requirements. Common electrolyte additives include sodium chloride (or acetate), potassium chloride (or acetate), calcium gluconate, magnesium sulfate, and sodium (or potassium) phosphate. Multiple vitamin preparations containing both water-soluble and fat-soluble vitamins are usually added on a daily basis. A trace element product containing zinc, copper, manganese, selenium, and chromium may be added.
IV fat emulsions	Intravenous fat (lipid) emulsion is required as a source of essential fatty acids. It is also used as a concentrated source of calories. Fat provides nine calories per gram, compared to 3.4 calories per gram provided by dextrose. Intravenous fat emulsion may be admixed into the parenteral nutrition solution with amino acids and dextrose, or piggybacked into the administration line.
peritoneal dialysis solutions	Used by patients who do not have functioning kidneys to remove toxic substances, excess body waste, and serum electrolytes through osmosis. The solution is administered directly into the peritoneal cavity (the cavity between the abdominal lining and the internal organs) to remove toxic substances, excess body waste, and serum electrolytes through osmosis. These solutions are hypertonic to blood so the water will not move into the circulatory system.

LAMINAR FLOW AND BIOLOGICAL SAFETY HOODS

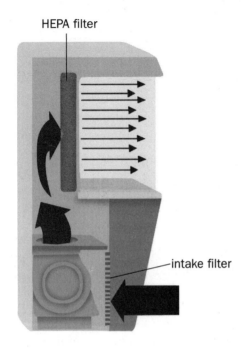

HEPA filter

intake filter

LAMINAR FLOW HOOD

With a Laminar flow hood, room air is drawn into a horizontal hood and passed through a prefilter to remove relatively large contaminants such as dust and lint. The air is then channeled through a high efficiency particulate air (HEPA) filter that removes particles larger than 0.3 μm (microns). The purified air then flows over the work surface in parallel lines at a uniform velocity (i.e., laminar flow). The constant flow of air from the hood prevents room air from entering the work area and removes contaminants introduced into the work area by material or personnel.

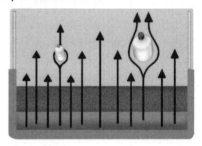

top down view

BIOLOGICAL SAFETY HOOD

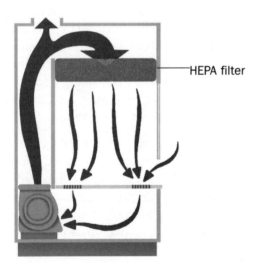

HEPA filter

Biological safety hoods protect both personnel and the environment from contamination. It is used in the preparation of hazardous drugs. A biological safety cabinet functions by passing air through a HEPA filter and directing it down toward the work area. As the air approaches the work surface, it is pulled through vents at the front, back, and sides of the hood. A major portion of the air is recirculated back into the cabinet and a minor portion passes through a secondary HEPA filter and is exhausted into the room.

RULES FOR WORKING WITH FLOW AND SAFETY HOODS

✔ **Never sneeze, cough, talk directly into a hood.**

✔ **Close doors or windows.** Breezes can disrupt the air flow sufficiently to contaminate the work area.

✔ **Perform all work at least 6 inches inside the hood** to derive the benefits of the laminar air flow. Laminar flow air begins to mix with outside air near the edge of the hood.

✔ **Maintain a direct, open path between the filter and the area inside the hood.**

✔ **Place nonsterile objects, such as solution containers or your hands, downstream from sterile ones.** Particles blown off these objects can contaminate anything downstream from them.

✔ **Do not put large objects at the back of the work area next to the filter.** They will disrupt air flow.

ASEPTIC TECHNIQUE

HAND WASHING

✔ Remove all jewelry and scrub hands and arms to the elbows with a suitable antibacterial agent.

✔ Stand far enough away from the sink so clothing does not come in contact with it.

✔ Turn on water. Wet hands and forearms thoroughly. Keep hands pointed downward.

✔ Scrub hands vigorously with an antibacterial soap.

✔ Work soap under fingernails by rubbing them against the palm of the other hand.

✔ Interlace the fingers and scrub the spaces between the fingers.

✔ Wash wrists and arms up to the elbows.

✔ Thoroughly rinse the soap from hands and arms.

✔ Dry hands and forearms thoroughly using a nonshedding paper towel.

✔ Use a dry paper towel to turn off the water faucet.

✔ After hands are washed, avoid touching clothes, face, hair, or any other potentially contaminated object in the area.

CLOTHING AND BARRIERS

✔ Wear clean lint-free garments or barrier clothing, including gowns, hair covers, and a mask.

✔ Wear sterile gloves.

✔ Follow facility or manufacturer guidelines for putting on and removing barrier clothing. Unless barriers are put on properly, they can easily become contaminated.

TRUE/FALSE

Indicate whether the statement is true or false in the blank. Answers are at the end of the book.

_____ 1. Pyrogens are a micronutrient in parenteral solutions.

_____ 2. 0.9% sodium chloride is an isotonic solution.

_____ 3. Physiological pH is about 7.4.

_____ 4. To practice aseptic technique, you must first sterilize your hands.

_____ 5. Fat provides 9 calories per gram, compared to 3.4 calories per gram provided by dextrose.

_____ 6. 5% dextrose is used as an irrigation solution.

EXPLAIN WHY

Explain why these statements are true or important. Check your answers in the text. Discuss any questions you may have with your Instructor.

1. Why should intravenous solutions generally be isotonic?

2. Why is the position of objects on a laminar flow hood work surface important?

3. Why is visual inspection of parenteral solutions important?

FILL IN THE KEY TERM

Answers are at the end of the book.

admixture	dialysis	hypotonic	osmolarity
ampules	diluent	infusion	osmosis
anhydrous	equivalent weight	ion	piggybacks
aseptic techniques	final filter	isotonic	pyrogens
bevel	flow rate	laminar flow	ready-to-mix systems
biological safety hoods	gauge	lumen	sharps
coring	HEPA filter	lyophilized	valence
coring	heparin lock	membrane filter	vial
depth filter	hypertonic	molecular weight	waters of hydration

1. _____ : Techniques that maintain sterile condition.

2. _____ : Chemicals produced by microorganisms that can cause pyretic (fever) reactions in patients.

3. _____ : A characteristic of a solution determined by the number of dissolved particles in it.

4. _____ : When a solution has an osmolarity equivalent to another.

5. _____ : When a solution has a greater osmolarity than another.

6. _____ : When a solution has a lesser osmolarity than another.

7. _____ : The rate (in ml/hour or ml/minute) at which the solution is administered to the patient.

8. _____ : An injection device which uses heparin to keep blood from clotting in the device.

9. _____ : Small volume solutions added to an LVP.

10. _____ : The slow continuous introduction of a solution into the blood stream.

11. _____ : The resulting solution when a drug is added to a parenteral solution.

12. _____ : Freeze-dried.

13. _____ : A liquid that dilutes a substance or solution.

14. _____ : Systems with predetermined amounts of admixture components for which admixing takes place just prior to administration.

15. _____ : An angled surface, as with the tip of a needle.

16. _____ : With needles, the higher the number, the thinner the lumen.

17. _____ : The hollow center of a needle.

18. _____ : When a needle damages the rubber closure of a parenteral container, causing fragments of the closure to fall into the container and contaminate its contents.

19. _____ : A filter that attaches to a syringe and filters solution through a membrane as the solution is expelled from the syringe.

20. _____ : A filter placed inside a needle hub that can filter solutions being drawn in or expelled, but not both.

21. _____ : A filter that filters solution immediately before it enters a patient's vein.

22. _____ : Continuous movement at a stable rate in one direction.

23. _____ : A high efficiency particulate air filter.

24. _____ : Are used in the preparation of hazardous drugs and protect both personnel and the environment from contamination.

25. _____ : A small glass or plastic container with a rubber closure sealing the contents in the container.

26. _____ : Sealed glass containers with an elongated neck that must be snapped off.

27. _____ : Needles, jagged glass or metal objects, or any items that might puncture or cut the skin.

28. _____ : A drug's molecular weight divided by its valence, a common measure of electrolytes.

29. _____ : The number of positive or negative charges on an ion.

30. _____ : The sum of the atomic weights of one molecule.

31. _____ : Molecular particles that carry electric charges.

32. _____ : Without water molecules.

33. _____ : Water molecules that attach to drug molecules.

34. _____ : The action in which drug in a higher concentration solution passes through a permeable membrane to a lower concentration solution.

35. _____ : Movement of particles in a solution through permeable membranes.

— 9 —

COMPOUNDING

KEY CONCEPTS

Test your knowledge by covering the information in the right hand column.

extemporaneous compounding	The on-demand preparation of a drug product according to a physician's prescription, formula, or recipe.
accuracy and stability	The supervising pharmacist must determine that a product can be accurately compounded and will be stable for its expected use. Accuracy is then essential in all weighings, measurements, and other activities in the compounding process.
class A balances	Can weigh as little as 120 mg of material with a 5% error. Always use the balance on a level surface and in a draft-free area. Always arrest the balance before adding or removing weight from either pan, or storing.
electronic or analytical balances	Highly sensitive balances that can weigh quantities smaller than 120 mg with acceptable accuracy.
weighing papers or boats	Should always be placed on the balance pans before any weighing is done. Balances must be readjusted after a new weighing paper or boat has been placed on each pan. Weighing papers taken from the same box can vary in weight by as much as 65 mg.
mortar and pestle	Made of three types of materials: glass, wedgewood; and porcelain. Wedgewood and porcelain mortars are used to grind crystals and large particles into fine powders. Glass mortars and pestles are preferable for mixing liquids and semi solid dosage forms.
volumetric glassware	For weighing liquid drugs, solvents, or additives. Includes graduates, flasks, pipets and syringes. Erlenmeyer flasks, beakers, and prescription bottles, regardless of markings, are not volumetric glassware.
small volumes	Always use the smallest device (graduate, pipet, syringe) that will accommodate the desired volume of liquid.

graduates	Cylindrical graduates are preferred over cone shaped because they are more accurate. When selecting a graduate, always choose the smallest graduate capable of containing the volume to be measured. Avoid measurements of volumes that are below 20 percent of the capacity of the graduate because the accuracy is unacceptable.
disposable syringe	Used to measure small volumes. Measurements made with syringes are more accurate and precise than those made with cylindrical graduates. Measure volumes to the edge of the syringe stopper.
meniscus	The curved surface of a volume of liquid. When reading a volume of a liquid against a graduation mark, hold the graduate so the meniscus is at eye level and read the mark at the bottom of the meniscus.
medicine droppers	Used to deliver small liquid doses, but must first be calibrated.
trituration	The fine grinding of a powder.
levigation	The trituration of a powdered drug with a solvent in which the drug is insoluble to reduce the particle size of the drug.
geometric dilution	A technique for mixing two powders of unequal size. The smaller amount of powder is diluted in steps by additions of the larger amount of powder.
solvents	Water is the most common solvent, but ethanol, glycerin, propylene glycol, or a variety of syrups may be used.
saturated solution	One that contains the maximum amount of drug it can accommodate at room temperature.
supersaturated solution	One that contains a larger amount of solute than it can normally accommodate at room temperature. Supersaturated solutions require heating.
syrup	A concentrated or nearly saturated solution of sucrose in water. Syrups containing flavoring agents are known as flavoring syrups (e.g. Cherry Syrup, Acacia Syrup, etc.). Medicinal syrups contain drugs (e.g. Guaifenesin Syrup). Syrup USP (sometimes referred to as Simple Syrup) contains 850 grams of sucrose and 450 ml of water in each liter of syrup. When fewer calories or sucrose properties are desired, syrups can be prepared from other sugars (e.g., glucose, fructose), non-sugar polyols (e.g., sorbitol, glycerin, propylene glycol, mannitol), or other non-nutritive artificial sweeteners (e.g., aspartame, saccharin).
elixirs	Hydroalcoholic solutions, i.e., they contain alcohol and water. The alcohol serves as the solvent for the drug.
thickening agents	Reduce the settling (sedimentation rate) of a suspension.

KEY CONCEPTS

Test your knowledge by covering the information in the right hand column.

suspensions	A "two-phase" compound consisting of a finely divided solid dispersed in a liquid. Most solid drugs are levigated in a mortar to reduce the particle size as much as possible before adding to the vehicle. Common levigating agents are alcohol or glycerin.
flocculating agents	Electrolytes that carry an electrical charge and enhance particle "dispersability" in a solution.
ointments and creams	Ointments are simple mixtures of a drug(s) in an ointment base. A cream is a semi-solid emulsion. Oleaginous (oil based) bases generally release substances slowly and unpredictably. Water miscible or aqueous bases tend to release drugs more rapidly.
emulsion	An unstable system consisting of at least two immiscible (unmixable) liquids, one that is dispersed as small droplets throughout the other, and a stabilizing agent.
oil-in-water (o/w)	An emulsion of oils, petroleum hydrocarbons, and/or waxes with water, where the aqueous phase is generally in excess of 45% of the total weight of the emulsion.
water-in-oil (w/o)	When water or aqueous solutions are dispersed in an oleaginous (oil based) medium, with the aqueous phase constituting less than 45% of the total weight.
emulsifiers	Emulsifiers provide a protective barrier around the dispersed droplets that stabilize the emulsion. Commonly used emulsifiers include: tragacanth, sodium lauryl sulfate, sodium dioctyl sulfosuccinate, and polymers known as the Spans and Tweens.
suppository bases	There are three classes that are based on their composition and physical properties: oleaginous bases, water soluble or miscible bases, and hydrophilic bases.
polyethylene glycols (PEGs)	Popular water soluble bases that are chemically stable, non-irritating, miscible with water and mucous secretions, and can be formulated by molding or compression in a wide range of hardnesses and melting points.
fusion molding	A method in which the drug is dispersed or dissolved in a melted suppository base. The fusion method can be used with all types of suppositories and must be used with most of them.
compression molding	A method of preparing suppositories by mixing the suppository base and the drug ingredients and forcing the mixture into a special compression mold.
capsules	When filling, the smallest capsule capable of containing the final volume is used since patients often have difficulty swallowing large capsules.

USING A BALANCE

Class A Balance

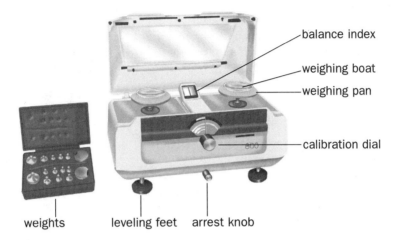

BASIC GUIDELINES FOR USING BALANCES

There are some general rules about using a balance that help to maintain the balance in top condition.

✔ Always cover both pans with weighing papers or use weighing boats. These protect the pans from abrasions, eliminate the need for repeated washing, and reduce loss of drug to porous surfaces.

✔ A clean paper or boat should be used for each new ingredient to prevent contamination of components.

✔ The balance must be readjusted after a new weighing paper or boat has been placed on each pan. Weighing papers taken from the same box can vary in weight by as much as 65 mg. If the new zero point is not established, an error of as much as 65 mg can be made. On 200 mg of material, this is more than 30%. Weighing boats also vary in weight.

✔ Always arrest the balance before adding or removing weight from either pan. Although the balance is noted for its durability, repeated jarring of the balance will ultimately damage the working mechanism of the balance and reduce its accuracy.

✔ Always clean the balance, close the lid, and arrest the pans before storing the balance between uses.

✔ Always use the balance on a level surface and in a draft-free area.

MEASURING

MENISCUS

When reading a volume of a liquid against a graduation mark, hold the graduate so the meniscus is at eye level and read the mark at the bottom of the meniscus. Viewing the level from above will create the incorrect impression that there is more volume in the graduate. If the container is very narrow, the meniscus can be quite large.

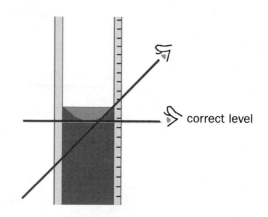

correct level

SYRINGE

When reading a volume of a liquid in a syringe, read to the edge of the stopper.

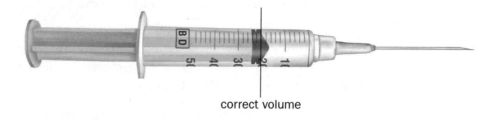

correct volume

CAPSULE SIZES

The relative sizes and fill capacities of capsules are:

Size	Volume (ml)
000	1.37
00	0.95
0	0.68
1	0.5
2	0.37
3	0.3
4	0.2
5	0.13

the punch method of filling capsules

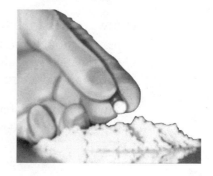

TRUE/FALSE

Indicate whether the statement is true or false in the blank. Answers are at the end of the book.

_____ 1. Compounding must always be done upon receipt of a prescription, never in advance.

_____ 2. Quantities smaller than 120 mg should be weighed on an electronic or analytical balance.

_____ 3. Cylindrical graduates are more accurate than conical ones.

_____ 4. Prescription bottles can be used as volumetric glassware.

_____ 5. Disposable syringes are generally used for measuring small volumes.

_____ 6. When aqueous and non aqueous solutions are mixed, the volume is always equal to the sum of the two volumes.

_____ 7. Levigation is the fine grinding of a powder.

_____ 8. Syrup USP is a supersaturated solution.

_____ 9. In elixirs, alcohol is the solvent for the drug.

_____ 10. With ointments, water miscible bases tend to release drugs more rapidly than oleaginous bases.

_____ 11. An emulsion containing 48% water would be a water-in-oil emulsion.

_____ 12. PEGs of different molecular weight are generally mixed to form a suppository base.

EXPLAIN WHY

Explain why these statements are true or important. Check your answers in the text. Discuss any questions you may have with your Instructor.

1. Why is the stability of a compound important?

2. Why is accuracy in each step of compounding important?

3. Why is the smallest device that will accommodate a volume used to measure it?

4. Why are class A balances not used for very small amounts?

5. Why is geometric dilution used when mixing unequal amounts of powders?

FILL IN THE KEY TERM

Answers are at the end of the book.

anticipatory com- pounding	extemporaneous com- pounding	meniscus	stability
		miscible	supersaturated solution
arrest knob	flocculating agent	mucilage	suspending agent
calibrate	fusion molding	oil-in-water	Syrup USP
compression molding	geometric dilution	primary emulsion	syrup
elixir	hydrophilic emulsifier	punch method	trituration
emulsifier	immiscible	saturated solution	volumetric
emulsion	levigation	solvents	water-in-oil
	lipophilic emulsifier	sonication	

1. _____ : The on-demand preparation of a drug product according to a physician's prescription, formula, or recipe.

2. _____ : The chemical and physical integrity of the dosage unit, and when appropriate, its ability to withstand microbiological contamination.

3. _____ : Compounding in advance of expected need.

4. _____ : To set, mark, or check the graduations of a measuring device.

5. _____ : Measures volume.

6. _____ : The knob on a balance that prevents any movement of the balance.

7. _____ : The curved surface of a column of liquid.

8. _____ : The fine grinding of a powder.

9. _____ : Triturating a powdered drug with a solvent in which it is insoluble to reduce its particle size.

10. _____ : A technique for mixing two powders of unequal size.

11. _____ : Exposure to high frequency sound waves.

12. _____ : Water is the most common, but ethanol, glycerin, propylene glycol, or a variety of syrups are used.

13. _____ : A solution containing the maximum amount of drug it can contain at room temperature.

14. _____ : A solution containing a larger amount of drug than it normally contains at room temperature.

15. _____ : A concentrated or nearly saturated solution of sucrose in water.

16. _____ : 850 grams of sucrose and 450 ml of water per liter.

17. _____ : Electrolytes used in the preparation of suspensions.

18. _____ : Hydroalcoholic solutions.

19. _____ : A thickening agent used in the preparation of suspensions.

20. _____ : Capable of being mixed together.

21. _____ : Cannot be mixed.

22. _____ : A stabilizing agent in emulsions.

23. _____ : An unstable system consisting of at least two immiscible liquids.

24. _____ : An emulsion in which water is dispersed through an oil base.

25. _____ : An emulsion in which oil is dispersed through a water base.

26. _____ : A stabilizing agent for water based dispersion mediums.

27. _____ : A stabilizing agent for oil based dispersion mediums.

28. _____ : The initial emulsion formed in a preparation to which ingredients are added to create the final volume.

29. _____ : A wet, slimy preparation formed as an initial step in a wet emulsion preparation method.

30. _____ : A method of making suppositories in which the ingredients are compressed in a mold.

31. _____ : A suppository preparation method in which the active ingredients are dispersed in a melted suppository base.

32. _____ : A method for filling capsules by repeatedly pushing or "punching" the capsule into an amount of drug powder.

STUDY NOTES

Use this area to write important points you'd like to remember.

— 10 —

BASIC BIOPHARMACEUTICS

KEY CONCEPTS

Test your knowledge by covering the information in the right hand column.

objective of drug therapy	To deliver the right drug, in the right concentration, to the right site of action at the right time to produce the desired effect.
receptors	When a drug produces an effect, it is interacting on a molecular level with cell material that is called a receptor. Receptor activation is responsible for most of the pharmacological responses in the body.
site of action	Only those drugs able to bind chemically to the receptors in a particular site of action can produce effects in that site. This is why specific cells only respond to certain drugs.
agonists	Drugs that activate receptors and produce a response that may either accelerate or slow normal cell processes.
antagonists	Drugs that bind to receptors but do not activate them. They prevent other drugs or substances from interacting with receptors.
dose-response curve	Specific doses of a drug is given to various subjects and the effect or response is measured in terms of dose and effect.
blood concentrations	The primary way to monitor a drug's concentration in the body and its related effect is to determine its blood concentrations.
minimum effective concentration (MEC)	When there is enough drug at the site of action to produce a response.
minimum toxic concentration (MTC)	An upper blood concentration limit beyond which there are undesired or toxic effects.

therapeutic window	The range between the minimum effective concentration and the minimum toxic concentration is called the therapeutic window. When concentrations are in this range, most patients receive the maximum benefit from their drug therapy with a minimum of risk.
ADME	Blood concentrations are the result of four simultaneously acting processes: absorption, distribution, metabolism, and excretion.
disposition	Another term for ADME.
elimination	Metabolism and excretion combined.
passive diffusion	Besides the four ADME processes, a critical factor of drug concentration and effect is how drugs move through biological membranes. Most drugs penetrate biological membranes by passive diffusion.
hydrophobic drugs	Lipid (fat) soluble drugs that penetrate the lipoidal (fat-like) cell membrane better than hydrophilic drugs.
hydrophilic drugs	Drugs that are attracted to water.
aqueous pores	Openings in cell membranes that allow entry of water and water soluble drugs.
absorption	The transfer of drug into the blood from an administered drug product is called absorption.
gastric emptying	Most drugs are given orally and absorbed into the blood from the small intestine. One of the primary factors affecting oral drug absorption is the gastric emptying time.
distribution	The movement of a drug within the body once the drug has reached the blood.
selective action	Drug action that is selective to certain tissues or organs, due both to the specific nature of receptor action as well as to various factors that can affect distribution.
protein binding	Many drugs bind to proteins in blood plasma to form a complex that is too large to penetrate cell openings. So the drug remains inactive.
metabolism	The body's process of transforming drugs. The primary site of drug metabolism in the body is the liver. Enzymes produced by the liver interact with drugs and transform them into metabolites.

enzyme	A complex protein that causes chemical reactions in other substances
metabolite	The transformed drug.
enzyme induction	The increase in enzyme activity that results in greater metabolism of drugs.
enzyme inhibition	The decrease in enzyme activity that results in reduced metabolism of drugs.
first-pass metabolism	When a drug is substantially degraded or destroyed by the liver's enzymes before it reaches the circulatory system, an important factor with orally administered drugs.
enterohepatic cycling	The transfer of drugs and their metabolites from the liver to the bile in the gall bladder and then into the intestine.
excretion	The process of excreting drugs and metabolites, primarily performed by the kidney through the urine.
glomerular filtration	The blood filtering process of the kidneys. As plasma water moves through the nephron, waste substances (including drugs and metabolites) are secreted into the fluid, with urine as the end result.
bioavailability	The amount of a drug that is available to the site of action and the rate at which it is available is called the bioavailability of the drug.
bioequivalents	Bioequivalent drug products are pharmaceutical equivalents or alternatives which have essentially the same rate and extent of absorption when administered at the same dose of the active ingredient under similar conditions.
pharmaceutical equivalents	Pharmaceutical equivalents are drug products that contain identical amounts of the same active ingredients in the same dosage form, but may contain different inactive ingredients.
pharmaceutical alternatives	Pharmaceutical alternatives are drug products that contain the identical active ingredients, but not necessarily in the same amount or dosage form.
therapeutic equivalent	Pharmaceutical equivalents that produce the same effects in patients.
therapeutic alternative	Drugs that have different active ingredients but produce similar therapeutic effects.

DOSE RESPONSE CURVE

When a series of specific doses is given to a number of people, the results show that some people respond to low doses but others require larger doses for a response to be produced. Some differences are due to the product itself, but most are due to human variability: different people have different characteristics that affect how a drug product behaves in them. A dose-response curve shows that as doses increase, responses increase up to a point where increased dosage no longer results in increased response.

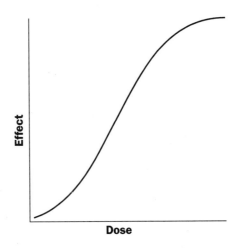

BLOOD CONCENTRATION—TIME PROFILES

Blood concentration begins at zero at the time the drug is administered (before it has been absorbed into the blood). With time, the drug leaves the formulation and enters the blood, causing concentrations to rise. Minimum effective concentration (MEC) is when there is enough drug at the site of action to produce a response. The time this occurs is called the onset of action. With most drugs, when blood concentrations increase, so does the intensity of the effect, since blood concentrations reflect the site of action concentrations that produce the response.

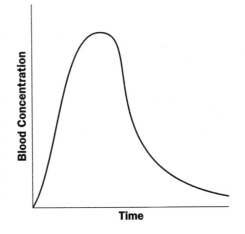

Some drugs have an upper blood concentration limit beyond which there are undesired or toxic effects. This limit is called the minimum toxic concentration (MTC). The range between the minimum effective concentration and the minimum toxic concentration is called the therapeutic window. When concentrations are in this range, most patients receive the maximum benefit from their drug therapy with a minimum of risk.

The last part of the curve shows the blood concentrations declining as absorption is complete. The time between the onset of action and the time when the minimum effective concentration is reached by the declining blood concentrations is called the duration of action. The duration of action is the time the drug should produce the desired effect.

ORAL ABSORPTION

Most drugs are given orally and absorbed into the blood from the small intestine. The small intestine's large surface area makes absorption easier. However, there are many conditions in the stomach that can affect absorption positively or negatively before the drug even reaches the small intestine. One of the primary factors affecting oral drug absorption is the gastric emptying time. This is the time a drug will stay in the stomach before it is emptied into the small intestine. Since stomach acid can degrade many drugs and since most absorption occurs in the intestine, gastric emptying time can significantly affect a drug's action. If a drug remains in the stomach too long, it can be degraded or destroyed, and its effect decreased. Gastric emptying time can be affected by a various conditions, including the amount and type of food in the stomach, the presence of other drugs, the person's body position, and their emotional condition. Some factors increase the gastric emptying time, but most slow it. The pH of the gastrointestinal organs is illustrated at right

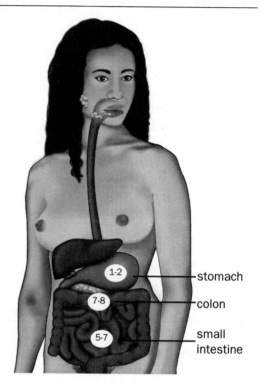

PASSIVE DIFFUSION

Before an effective concentration of a drug can reach its site of action, it must overcome many barriers, most of which are biological membranes, complex structures composed of lipids (fats) and proteins. Most drugs penetrate biological membranes by passive diffusion. This occurs when drugs in the body's fluids move from an area of higher concentration to an area of lower concentration, until the concentrations in each area are in a state of equilibrium. Passive diffusion causes most orally administered drugs to move from the intestine to the blood and from the blood to the site of action.

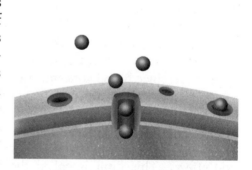

PROTEIN BINDING

Many drugs bind to proteins in blood plasma to form a complex that is too large to penetrate cell openings. So the drug remains inactive. Protein binding can be considered a type of drug storage within the body. Some drugs bind extensively to proteins in fat and muscle, and are gradually released as the blood concentration of the drug falls. These drugs remain in the body a long time, and therefore have a long duration of action.

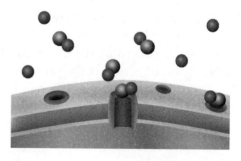

TRUE/FALSE

Indicate whether the statement is true or false in the blank. Answers are at the end of the book.

_____ 1. Receptors are located on the surfaces of cell membranes and inside cells.

_____ 2. Agonists may produce a response that slows normal cell process.

_____ 3. Antagonists bind to cell receptors but do not activate them.

_____ 4. After all receptors are occupied by a drug, its effect can still be increased by increasing the dose.

_____ 5. The number or sensitivity of receptors is not affected by prolonged drug use.

_____ 6. Most patients receive the maximum benefit from drug therapy when the amount of the drug in the blood is between the minimum effective and minimum toxic concentration.

_____ 7. Passive diffusion is the most common way an orally administered drug is distributed through the body.

_____ 8. Cell membranes generally absorb hydrophilic drugs more easily than hydrophobic ones.

_____ 9. Most orally administered drugs are absorbed from the stomach.

_____ 10. Protein binding can result in the gradual release of a drug into the bloodstream.

_____ 11. Most drugs and metabolites are excreted by the liver.

EXPLAIN WHY

Explain why these statements are true or important. Check your answers in the text. Discuss any questions you may have with your Instructor.

1. Why can a drug be developed to have a specific therapeutic effect?

2. Why can the same drug have different effects in different people?

3. Why is gastric emptying time important?

4. Why does the chronic administration of some drugs require increases in dosage to achieve the same effect or decreases to avoid toxicity?

5. Why is a pharmaceutical equivalent not necessarily therapeutically equivalent?

FILL IN THE KEY TERM

Answers are at the end of the book.

active transport
agonist
antagonist
bioavailability
bioequivalence
biopharmaceutics
complex
disposition
enterohepatic cycling
enzyme

enzyme induction
enzyme inhibition
first pass metabolism
gastric emptying time
glomerular filtration
hydrophilic
hydrophobic
lipoidal
metabolite
minimum effective concentration
nephron

onset of action
passive diffusion
pharmaceutical alternative
pharmaceutical equivalent
protein binding
receptor
selective action
site of action
therapeutic equivalent
therapeutic window

1. _____ : The study of the factors associated with drug products and physiological processes, and the resulting systemic concentrations of the drugs.

2. _____ : The location where an administered drug produces an effect.

3. _____ : The cellular material at the site of action which interacts with the drug.

4. _____ : The characteristic of a drug that makes its action specific to certain receptors and the tissues they affect.

5. _____ : Drugs that activate receptors to accelerate or slow normal cell function.

6. _____ : Drugs that bind with receptors but do not activate them. They block receptor action by preventing other drugs or substances from activating them.

7. _____ : The blood concentration needed of a drug to produce a response.

8. _____ : The time MEC is reached and the response occurs.

9. _____ : A drug's blood concentration range between its minimum effective concentration and minimum toxic concentration.

10. _____ : A term sometimes used to refer to all of the ADME processes together.

11. _____ : The movement of drugs from an area of higher concentration to lower concentration.

12. _____ : The movement of drug molecules across membranes by active means, rather than passive diffusion.

13. _____ : Water repelling; cannot associate with water.

14. _____ : Capable of associating with or absorbing water.

15. _____ : Fat like substance.

16. _____ : The time a drug will stay in the stomach before it is emptied into the small intestine.

17. _____ : Formed when molecules of different chemicals attach to each other, as in protein binding.

18. _____ : The attachment of a drug molecule to a plasma or tissue protein, effectively making the drug inactive, but also keeping it within the body.

19. _____ : The substance resulting from the body's transformation of an administered drug.

20. _____ : A complex protein that causes chemical reactions in other substances.

21. _____ : The increase in enzyme activity that results in greater metabolism of drugs.

22. _____ : The decrease in enzyme activity that results in reduced metabolism of drugs.

23. _____ : The substantial degradation of a drug caused by enzyme metabolism in the liver before the drug reaches the systemic circulation.

24. _____ : The transfer of drugs and their metabolites from the liver to the bile in the gall bladder and then into the intestine.

25. _____ : The functional unit of the kidneys.

26. _____ : The blood filtering process of the kidneys.

27. _____ : The relative amount of an administered dose that reaches the general circulation and the rate at which this occurs.

28. _____ : The comparison of bioavailability between two dosage forms.

29. _____ : Drug products that contain identical amounts of the same active ingredients in the same dosage form.

30. _____ : Drug products that contain the same active ingredients, but not necessarily in the same amount or dosage form.

31. _____ : Pharmaceutical equivalents that produce the same effects in patients.

— 11 —

FACTORS AFFECTING DRUG ACTIVITY

KEY CONCEPTS

Test your knowledge by covering the information in the right hand column.

human variability	Differences in age, weight, genetics, and gender are among the significant factors that influence the differences in medication responses among people.
age	Drug distribution, metabolism, and excretion are quite different in the neonate and infant than in adults because their organ systems are not fully developed. Children metabolize certain drugs more rapidly than adults. The elderly typically consume more drugs than other age groups. They also experience physiological changes that significantly affect drug action.
pregnancy	A number of physiological changes that occur in women in the latter stages of pregnancy tend to reduce the rate of absorption.
genetics	Genetic differences can cause differences in the types and amounts of proteins produced in the body, which can result in differences in drug action.
weight	Weight adjustments may be needed for individuals whose weight is more than 50% higher than the average adult weight. Weight adjustments are also made for children, or unusually small, emaciated, or obese adult patients.
allergic reactions	Almost any drug, in almost any dose, can produce an allergic or hypersensitive reaction in a patient. Anaphylactic shock is a potentially fatal hypersensitivity reaction.
common adverse reactions	Anorexia, nausea, vomiting, constipation, and diarrhea are among the most common adverse reactions to drugs.
teratogenicity	The ability of a substance to cause abnormal fetal development when given to pregnant women.

drug-drug interactions	These can result in either increases or decreases in therapeutic effects or adverse effects.
additive effects	Occur when two drugs with similar pharmacological actions are taken, e.g., alcohol and a sedative together produce increased sedation.
synergism or potentiation	Occurs when two drugs with different sites or mechanisms of action produce greater effects when taken together than either does when taken alone, e.g., acetaminophen and codeine together produce increased analgesia.
interference	One drug can interfere with the elimination of a second drug and intensify the effects of the second drug, e.g., cimetidine inhibits metabolizing enzymes and therefore the metabolism and elimination of many drugs.
displacement	Displacement of one drug from protein binding sites by a second drug increases the effects of the displaced drug. Decreased intestinal absorption can occur when orally taken drugs combine to produce nonabsorbable compounds, e.g.. when magnesium hydroxide and oral tetracyline bind.
enzyme induction	Caused when drugs activate metabolizing enzymes in the liver, increasing the metabolism of other drugs affected by the same enzymes.
increased excretion	Some drugs raise urinary pH, lessening renal reabsorption, e.g., sodium bicarbonate raises pH and will cause increased elimination of phenobarbital.
drug-diet interactions	The physical presence of food in the gastrointestinal tract can alter absorption by interacting chemically (e.g., certain medications and tetracycline); improving the water-solubility of some drugs by increasing bile secretion; affecting the performance of the dosage form (e.g., altering the release characteristics of polymer-coated tablets); altering gastric emptying; altering intestinal movement; altering liver blood flow. Some foods contain substances that react with certain drugs, e.g., foods containing tyramine can react with monoamine oxidase (MAO) inhibitors.
disease states	The disposition and effect of some drugs can be influenced by the presence of diseases other than the one for which a drug is used. Hepatic, cardiovascular, renal, and endocrine disease all increase the variability in drug response. For example, decreased blood flow from cardiovascular disorders can delay or cause erratic drug absorption.

FILL IN THE KEY TERM

Answers are at the end of the book.

acute viral hepatitis	displacement	hypothyroidism
additive effects	drug-diet interactions	idiosyncrasy
anaphylactic shock	hepatic disease	interference
antidote	hepatotoxity	nephrotoxicity
carcinogenicity	hypersensitivity	synergism
cirrhosis	hyperthyroidism	teratogenicity

1. _____ : An abnormal sensitivity generally resulting in an allergic reaction.

2. _____ : A potentially fatal hypersensitivity reaction producing severe respiratory distress and cardiovascular collapse.

3. _____ : An unexpected reaction the first time a drug is taken, generally due to genetic causes.

4. _____ : Toxicity of the liver.

5. _____ : The ability of a substance to harm the kidneys.

6. _____ : The ability of a substance to cause cancer.

7. _____ : The ability of a substance to cause abnormal fetal development when given to pregnant women.

8. _____ : The increase in effect when two drugs with similar pharmacological actions are taken.

9. _____ : When two drugs with different sites or mechanisms of action produce greater effects when taken together than when taken alone.

10. _____ : When one drug interferes with the elimination of a second drug and intensify the effects of the second drug.

11. _____ : When one drug is moved from protein binding sites by a second drug, resulting in increased effects of the displaced drug.

12. _____ : A drug that antagonizes the toxic effect of another drug.

13. _____ : When elements of ingested nutrients interact with a drug and this affects the disposition of the drug.

14. _____ : A condition in which thyroid hormone secretions are below normal, often referred to as an underactive thyroid.

15. _____ : A condition in which thyroid hormone secretions are above normal, often referred to as an overactive thyroid.

16. _____ : Liver disease.

17. _____ : A chronic and potentially fatal liver disease causing loss of function and resistance to blood flow through the liver.

18. _____ : A virally caused systemic infection that causes inflammation of the liver.

TRUE/FALSE

Indicate whether the statement is true or false in the blank. Answers are at the end of the book.

_____ 1. Human variability is not a significant factor in disposition.

_____ 2. Infants are not able to eliminate drugs as efficiently as adults.

_____ 3. Lower cardiac output in the elderly tends to slow the distribution of drugs.

_____ 4. Commonly used drugs such as acetaminophen and aspirin can produce hepatotoxicity.

_____ 5. Ibuprofen can cause nephrotoxicity.

_____ 6. Analgesics and antihistamines are not considered teratogenic.

_____ 7. Some anticancer drugs are considered carcinogenic.

_____ 8. If one drug interferes with the elimination of another, the effects of the other drug will be decreased.

_____ 9. If one drug displaces another from a protein binding site, the effects of the displaced drug increase.

_____ 10. Cigarette smoking can cause enzyme induction.

EXPLAIN WHY

Explain why these statements are true or important. Check your answers in the text. Discuss any questions you may have with your Instructor.

1. Give at least three reasons why drug-drug interactions can increase the effects of drugs.

2. Give at least three reasons why drug-drug interactions can decrease the effects of drugs.

3. Give at least three reasons diet can affect drug activity.

— 12 —

INFORMATION

KEY CONCEPTS

Test your knowledge by covering the information in the right hand column.

primary literature	Information based directly on contemporary research.
secondary literature	Primarily general reference works based upon primary literature sources.
tertiary literature	Condensed and compact information based on primary literature.
abstracting services	Services that summarize information from various primary sources for quick reference.
Material Safety Data Sheets (MSDS)	OSHA required information for handling hazardous chemicals.
state regulations	Many states have laws or State Board of Pharmacy rules and regulations that require pharmacies to maintain specific professional literature references.
Drug Facts and Comparisons (DFC)	A preferred reference for comprehensive and timely drug information, containing information about prescription and OTC products.
Martindale	"The Extra Pharmacopoeia," the best source of information on drugs in clinical use internationally.
Physician's Desk Reference	An annual publication intended for physicians that provides prescription information on major pharmaceutical products.
American Hospital Formulary Service	The authority for drug information questions. It groups drug monographs by therapeutic use.
USP DI	Provides comprehensive and clinically relevant information on drugs in current use.

Handbook on Injectable Drugs	A collection of monographs on commercially available parenteral drugs that include concentration, stability, dosage and compatibility information.
Merck Index	An encyclopedic source of chemical substance data, contains monographs referenced by trade, code, chemical, investigational and abbreviated drug names.
American Drug Index	An exhaustive list of drug products and contains trade and generic drug names, phonetic pronunciations, indications, manufacturers and schedule information in a dictionary format.
Drug Topics Red Book and American Druggist Blue Book	The pharmacist's guides to products and prices, providing annual price lists of drug products including manufacturer, package size, strength and wholesale and retail prices.
"Orange Book"	The common name for the FDA's Approved Drug Products publication.
Internet	A "supernetwork" of many networks from around the world all connected to each other by telephone lines, and all using a common "language."
search engine	Internet software that searches the Web for specific information you enter.
URLs (uniform resource locators)	The specific addresses of Web sites you want to visit.

STUDY NOTES

Use this area to write important points or Web addresses you'd like to remember.

FILL IN THE KEY TERM

Answers are at the end of the book.

abstracting services
American Hospital Formulary
   Service
browser
Drug Facts and Comparisons

Handbook on Injectable
   Drugs
Internet Service Provider (ISP)
Material Safety Data Sheets
modem
primary literature

secondary literature
tertiary literature
URL
USP DI
World Wide Web

1. _____ : Original reports of clinical and other types of research projects and studies.

2. _____ : Condensed works based on primary literature, such as textbooks, monographs, etc.

3. _____ : Services that summarize information from various primary sources for quick reference.

4. _____ : OSHA required information for handling hazardous chemicals.

5. _____ : General reference works based upon primary literature sources.

6. _____ : The authority for drug information questions. It groups drug monographs by therapeutic use.

7. _____ : A preferred reference for comprehensive and timely drug information, containing information about prescription and OTC products.

8. _____ : Provides comprehensive and clinically relevant information on drugs in current use.

9. _____ : A collection of monographs on commercially available parenteral drugs that include concentration, stability, dosage and compatibility information.

10. _____ : A collection of electronic documents at addresses called Web sites.

11. _____ : A piece of hardware that enables a computer to communicate through telephone lines.

12. _____ : A software program that allows users to view Web sites on the World Wide Web.

13. _____ : A company that provides access to the Internet.

14. _____ : A web address.

TRUE/FALSE

Indicate whether the statement is true or false in the blank. Answers are at the end of the book.

_____ 1. Primary literature is the largest but least current source of information.

_____ 2. MSDS's provide information on the proper protective measures for exposure to hazardous chemicals.

_____ 3. Drug Facts and Comparisons provides information on prescription and OTC drug products, divided into therapeutic groups.

_____ 4. AHSF is a collection of monographs on parenteral drugs.

_____ 5. The PDR is revised once every two years.

_____ 6. The "Orange Book" is included in Volume III of the USP DI: Approved Drug Products and Legal Requirements.

_____ 7. MEDLINE is an annual publication of international medical literature.

_____ 8. The Handbook of Nonprescription Drugs is a comprehensive source of information on OTC products.

_____ 9. A modem is software that allows you to view web sites.

_____ 10. AltaVista is an Internet search engine.

_____ 11. Certified technicians (CPhTs) must obtain 20 hours of continuing education credits every two years to maintain certification.

EXPLAIN WHY

Explain why these statements are true or important. Check your answers in the text. Discuss any questions you may have with your Instructor.

1. Why is primary literature important?

2. Why is continuing education important?

3. Why should technicians be familiar with pharmaceutical information sources?

4. Why should you know how to use an Internet search engine?

— 13 —

INVENTORY MANAGEMENT

KEY CONCEPTS

Test your knowledge by covering the information in the right hand column.

inventory goals	Good inventory management ensures that drugs which are likely to be needed are both on hand and usable—that is, not expired, damaged, contaminated, or otherwise unfit for use.
open formulary	One that allows purchase of any medication that is prescribed.
closed formulary	A limited list of approved medications.
wholesalers	More than three-quarters of pharmaceutical manufacturers' sales are directly to drug wholesalers, who in turn resell their inventory to hospitals, pharmacies, and other pharmaceutical dispensers. They are government-licensed and regulated.
Schedule II substances	Must be stocked separately in a secure place and require a special order form for reordering. Their stock must be continually monitored and documented.
perpetual inventory	A system that maintains a continuous record of every item in inventory so that it always shows the stock on hand.
spoilage	Inappropriate storage conditions or expired products automatically determine that a product is spoiled since in either case the chemical compounds in the drug product may have degraded.
turnover	The rate at which inventory is used.
point of sale (POS) system	A system in which the item is deducted from inventory as it is sold or dispensed.
drug reorder points	Maximum and minimum inventory levels for each drug.
hard copy	Important reports (especially purchase orders) should be regularly printed out and filed as hard copy both for convenience and as a backup record-keeping system.

computer maintenance	Factors that can damage computer systems are temperature, dust, moisture, movement, vibrations, and power surges.
data back-up	Pharmacy computer files must be regularly backed-up or copied to an appropriate storage media.
order entry device	In a computerized inventory system, a hand-held device to generate orders.
online ordering	In an online ordering system, if an order can be filled as ordered, a message from the supplier will automatically confirm the order to the ordering system. The system automatically assigns to each order a purchase order number for identification.
Material Safety Data Sheets	Instructions for hazardous substances such as chemotherapeutic agents that indicate when special handling and shipping is required.
controlled substance shipping	These substances are shipped separately and checked in by a pharmacist. A special order form must be used for Schedule II substances.
stock bottles	The bulk containers in which most medications are received from the supplier.
storage	Drugs must be stored according to manufacturer's specifications. Most drugs are kept in a fairly constant room temperature of 59°-86°F. The temperature of refrigeration should generally be 36°-46°.
freshness	Medications should be organized in a way that will dispense the oldest items first.
dispensing units	In hospitals and other settings, medications are stocked in dispensing units throughout the facility that may be called supply stations or med-stations.

STUDY NOTES

Use this area to write important points you'd like to remember.

FILL IN THE KEY TERM

Answers are at the end of the book.

closed formulary   order entry device   Schedule II substances
database   perpetual inventory   stock bottles
dispensing units   point of sale system   turnover
open formulary   purchase order number   unit-dose
                       reorder points

1. _____ : One that allows purchase of any medication that is prescribed.

2. _____ : A limited list of approved medications.

3. _____ : The rate at which inventory is used, generally expressed in number of days.

4. _____ : Must be stocked separately in a secure place and require a special order form for reordering. Their stock must be continually monitored and documented.

5. _____ : A system that maintains a continuous record of every item in inventory so that it always shows the stock on hand.

6. _____ : An inventory system in which the item is deducted from inventory as it is sold or dispensed.

7. _____ : Minimum and maximum stock levels which determine when a reorder is placed and for how much.

8. _____ : In a computerized inventory system, a hand-held device to generate orders.

9. _____ : A collection of information structured so that specific information within it can easily be retrieved and used.

10. _____ : A number assigned to each order for products that will allow it to tracked and checked throughout the order process.

11. _____ : The bulk containers in which most medications are received from the supplier.

12. _____ : A package containing a single dose of a medication.

13. _____ : In hospitals and other settings, medications are stocked in units throughout the facility that may also be called supply stations or med-stations.

TRUE/FALSE

Indicate whether the statement is true or false in the blank. Answers are at the end of the book.

_____ 1. The majority of pharmaceutical manufacturer sales are to wholesalers.

_____ 2. Drug products can always be sold right up to their date of expiration.

_____ 3. Reorder points are maximum and minimum inventory levels for a product.

_____ 4. Computerized ordering systems do not allow manual editing.

_____ 5. Computers can be adversely affected by dust.

_____ 6. With computers keeping records, printed copies are not needed.

_____ 7. Certain hazardous substances may not be shipped by air.

_____ 8. Schedule II substances may be stored with non-controlled substances.

_____ 9. Most drug products should be stored at 50°-59°.

_____ 10. Hospitals frequently use drug dispensing units located at points of use throughout the hospital.

EXPLAIN WHY

Explain why these statements are true or important. Check your answers in the text. Discuss any questions you may have with your Instructor.

1. Why are wholesalers used?

2. Why is knowing the turnover rate of a product important?

3. Why are reorder points used?

4. Why is it important to make hard copy of computerized reports?

5. Why is it important to back up computer files?

— 14 —

FINANCIAL ISSUES

KEY CONCEPTS

Test your knowledge by covering the information in the right hand column.

third party programs
Another party besides the patient or the pharmacy that pays for some or all of the cost of medication: essentially, an insurer.

pharmacy benefit manager (PBM)
A company that administers drug benefit programs for insurance companies, HMOs, and self-insured employers.

co-insurance
Essentially an agreement between the insurer and the insured to share costs.

co-pay
The portion of the cost of prescriptions that patients with third party insurance must pay.

deductible
A set amount that must be paid by the patient for each benefit period before the insurer will cover additional expenses.

maximum allowable cost (MAC)
The amount paid by the insurer is not equal to the retail price normally charged, but is determined by a formula described in a contract between the insurer and the pharmacy. There is a maximum allowable cost (MAC) per tablet or other dispensing unit that an insurer or PBM will pay for a given product.

usual and customary (U&C)
The MAC is often determined by survey of the usual and customary (U&C) prices for a prescription within a given geographic area. This is also referred to as the UCR (usual, customary, and reasonable) price for the prescription.

prescription drug benefit cards
Cards that contain necessary billing information for pharmacies, including the patient's identification number, group number, and co-pay amount.

HMO (health maintenance organization)
Health care networks that usually do not cover expenses incurred outside the network and often require generic substitution.

POS (point of service)	Health care network where the patient's primary care physician must be a member and costs outside the network may be partially reimbursed.
PPO (preferred provider organization)	Health care network that reimburses expenses outside the network at a lower rate than inside the network and usually requires generic substitution.
workers' compensation	Compensation for employees accidentally injured on-the-job.
Medicare	National health insurance for people over the age of 65, disabled people under the age of 65, and people with kidney failure.
Medicaid	A federal-state program for the needy.
online adjudication	Most prescription claims are now filed electronically by online claim submission and online adjudication of claims. In online adjudication, the technician uses the computer to determine the exact coverage for each prescription with the appropriate third party.
dispense as written	When brand name drugs are dispensed, numbers corresponding to the reason for submitting the claim with brand name drugs are entered in a DAW (dispense as written) indicator field in the prescription system.
patient identification number	The number assigned to the patient by the insurer that is indicated on the drug benefit card. If it does not match the code for the patient in the insurer's computer (with the same sex and other information) a claim may be rejected.
age limitations	Many prescription drug plans have age limitations for children or dependents of the cardholder.
refills	Most third party plans require that most of the medication has been taken before the plan will cover a refill of the same medication.
maintenance medications	Many managed care health programs require mail order pharmacies to fill prescriptions for maintenance medications.
rejected claims	When a claim is rejected, the pharmacy technician can telephone the insurance plan's pharmacy help desk to determine if the patient is eligible for coverage.
audits	Pharmacy benefits managers audit pharmacies to confirm that their billing practices are proper.

FILL IN THE KEY TERM

Answers are at the end of the book.

co-insurance
co-pay
deductible
dual co-pay
HMOs
maximum allowable cost (MAC)

Medicaid
Medicare
online adjudication
patient assistance programs
patient identification number
pharmacy benefits managers
POSs

PPOs
prescription drug benefit cards
Qualified Medicare Beneficiaries
U&C or UCR
universal claim form
workers' compensation

1. _____ : Companies that administer drug benefit programs.

2. _____ : The resolution of prescription coverage through the communication of the pharmacy computer with the third party computer.

3. _____ : An agreement for cost-sharing between the insurer and the insured.

4. _____ : The portion of the price of medication that the patient is required to pay.

5. _____ : Co-pays that have two prices: one for generic and one for brand medications.

6. _____ : The maximum price per tablet (or other dispensing unit) an insurer or PBM will pay for a given product.

7. _____ : The maximum amount of payment for a given prescription, determined by the insurer to be a reasonable price.

8. _____ : A network of providers for which costs are covered inside but not outside of the network.

9. _____ : A network of providers where the patient's primary care physician must be a member and costs outside the network may be partially reimbursed.

10. _____ : A network of providers where costs outside the network may be partially reimbursed and the patient's primary care physician need not be a member.

11. _____ : A set amount that must be paid by the patient for each benefit period before the insurer will cover additional expenses.

12. _____ : Cards that contain third party billing information for prescription drug purchases.

13. _____ : The number assigned to the patient by the insurer that is indicated on the drug benefit card.

14. _____ : A federal program providing health care to people with certain disabilities over age 65.

15. _____ : A federal-state program, administered by the states, providing health care for the needy.

16. _____ : Medicare patients who may at times qualify for prescription drug coverage through a state administered program.

17. _____ : An employer compensation program for employees accidentally injured on the job.

18. _____ : Manufacturer sponsored prescription drug programs for the needy.

19. _____ : A standard claim form accepted by many insurers.

TRUE/FALSE

Indicate whether the statement is true or false in the blank. Answers are at the end of the book.

_____ 1. The amount paid by a co-insurer to the pharmacy is equal to the wholesale price of a drug.

_____ 2. In online adjudication, the claim processing computer determines if the claim is valid and what the co-pay should be, usually in less than a minute.

_____ 3. A pharmacy benefits manager is a company that administers drug benefits programs.

_____ 4. A dual co-pay means that the patient will pay a different co-pay for generic and brand drugs.

_____ 5. It is up to the pharmacist to decide if generic substitution is available.

_____ 6. HMOs often require that prescriptions for maintenance medications be filled by a mail order pharmacy.

_____ 7. All Medicaid programs have an open formulary.

_____ 8. An NABP number identifies the pharmacy.

EXPLAIN WHY

Explain why these statements are true or important. Check your answers in the text. Discuss any questions you may have with your Instructor.

1. If an online claim is rejected, why is it important to review the information that was originally entered before calling?

2. Why is it important to know the benefits of various third party programs?

— 15 —

COMMUNITY PHARMACY

KEY CONCEPTS

Test your knowledge by covering the information in the right hand column.

community pharmacy

The pharmacy practice that provides prescription services to the public. In addition to prescription drugs, community pharmacies sell over-the-counter medications as well as other health and beauty products. In the United States, more than half of all prescription drugs are dispensed by community pharmacies. There are about 60,000 community pharmacies.

counseling

The role of the community pharmacist in counseling and educating patients has been steadily increasing. In the United States, the 1990 Omnibus Budget and Reconciliation Act (OBRA) required community pharmacists to offer counseling to Medicaid patients regarding medications. Many states have expanded this requirement to apply to all customers.

regulation

Community pharmacies are most closely regulated at the state level. In addition to the many regulations on prescribers and prescriptions, states regulations include such things as the ratio of pharmacists to technicians, scope of practice, record keeping, equipment, and work areas.

customer service

A major area of importance in the community pharmacy, since technicians constantly interact with patients as customers. It is important to always respond to customers in a positive and courteous way.

interpersonal skills

Skills involving relationships between people. Good interpersonal skills are based on techniques such as looking the other person in the eye, listening carefully , etc.

telephone use

Telephone calls must be answered in a pleasant and courteous manner, following a standard format that should be indicated by the store manager or pharmacist.

refills	When processing a refill prescription, it is necessary to check that there are refills available. In the case of a patient requesting an early refill of a controlled substance, involve the pharmacist right away.
drug interactions	Whenever the prescription system flags drug interactions and allergy conflicts, alert the pharmacist so that he or she can evaluate the significance of the flag.
safety caps	All dispensed prescription vials and bottles must have a safety cap or child resistant cap, unless the patient requests an easy-open or non-child resistant cap.
auxiliary labels	Auxiliary labels identify important usage information, including specific warnings or alerts on: administration, proper storage, possible side effects, and potential food and drug interactions.
final check by pharmacist	As a final step of the prescription preparation process, the final product and all paperwork, including the original prescription, is organized for the pharmacist's final check.
signature log	Customer signatures in a log are required for Medicaid and most third party insurer or HMO prescriptions, along with Schedule V controlled substances, poisons, and certain other prescriptions (depending upon the state).
mark-up	The amount of the retailer's sale price minus their purchase price. It is calculated by multiplying the retailer's purchase price by the mark-up percentage. For example, a 30% mark-up on an item purchased for $2.30 is $0.69 (2.30 x 0.3), so the sale price would be $2.99.
OTC products	Drug products that do not require a prescription, but are not without risks. Therefore, the technician should not recommend them to pharmacy customers.
shelf stickers	Stickers for OTC drugs and other products that can be scanned for inventory identification.
unit price	The price of a single unit of a product, such as for one ounce of a liquid cold remedy.
stickering	Technicians often apply prices to products using a stickering gun or by hand.
stock	Managing stock is often a technician responsibility and includes ordering, receiving, storing, and placing products on shelves.

FILL IN THE KEY TERM

Answers are at the end of the book.

auxiliary labels	group number	safety caps
bar code	interpersonal skills	signa
confidentiality	OBRA '90	scope of practice
counting tray	patient identification number	shelf stickers
DEA number	refrigeration	unit price

1. _____ : Required community pharmacists to offer counseling to Medicaid patients regarding medications.

2. _____ : Based on techniques such as looking the other person in the eye, listening carefully, etc.

3. _____ : What technicians may and may not do, as mandated by their state.

4. _____ : The requirement to keep patient information private between the patient and the patient's care providers.

5. _____ : Temperature should be between 2°-8° C (36°-46°F).

6. _____ : The number of the patient's insurance policy as indicated on their drug benefit card.

7. _____ : A number that identifies a patient's employer.

8. _____ : Directions for use.

9. _____ : Required for all controlled substance prescriptions and by many third party insurers.

10. _____ : Child resistant caps required of all dispensed prescription vials.

11. _____ : A tray designed for counting pills.

12. _____ : Stickers with product information that can be scanned for inventory identification.

13. _____ : A series of lines that identify a product when scanned.

14. _____ : Labels regarding specific warnings and usage information.

15. _____ : For example, the price for one ounce of a liquid cold remedy.

TRUE/FALSE

Indicate whether the statement is true or false in the blank. Answers are at the end of the book.

_____ 1.   More than half of all drugs in the U.S. are sold at community pharmacies.

_____ 2.   Many states put limits on the number of technicians assisting the pharmacist at a given time.

_____ 3.   It is important to get the prescription number for refills.

_____ 4.   The DAW code is only required for controlled substance prescriptions.

_____ 5.   It is up to the pharmacist to decide the number of refills.

_____ 6.   Safety caps are not used for patients who request an easy open cap.

_____ 7.   When the computerized prescription system flags a drug interaction or allergy, the person to tell this to is the patient.

_____ 8.   When a technician prepares a prescription, it is always checked by the pharmacist before dispensing to the patient.

_____ 9.   Medicaid requires signatures for dispensed prescriptions.

_____ 10. OTC products may be purchased without a prescription because they are without risk.

_____ 11. Expired drugs must either be returned to the wholesaler or destroyed.

EXPLAIN WHY

Explain why these statements are true or important. Check your answers in the text. Discuss any questions you may have with your Instructor.

1. Why is the health of customers a factor in community pharmacy?

2. Why are good interpersonal skills important in community pharmacy?

3. Why is it important to look a patient in the eye and restate what they have said?

4. Why does the pharmacist check technician filled prescriptions before dispensing to patients?

5. Why shouldn't technicians recommend OTC products?

— 16 —

INSTITUTIONAL PHARMACY

KEY CONCEPTS

Test your knowledge by covering the information in the right hand column.

24-hour care	Hospitals provide care around the clock. Standard shifts are 7am to 3:30pm; 3:00pm to 11:30pm; and 11:00pm to 7:00am.
patient care units	Patient rooms are divided into groups called nursing units or patient care units, with patients having similar problems often located on the same unit.
nurse's station	The work station for medical personnel on a nursing unit is called the nurse's station. Various items required for care of patients are stored there, including patient medications.
ancillary areas	Areas such as the emergency room that also use medications and are serviced by the pharmacy department.
pharmacist supervision	Pharmacy technicians in the hospital work under the direct supervision of a pharmacist. Only a pharmacist may verify orders in the computer system and check medications being sent to the nursing floors.
patient drug profiles	Computer generated drug profiles are prepared daily for each patient
patient medication trays	The amount of medications for a 24 hour period are placed in patient trays that are loaded into medication carts.
unit doses	The amount of drug required for one dose, called a unit dose.
unit dose labels	Unit dose labels contain bar codes for identification and control. Items are scanned into the dispensing and inventory system at various stages up to dispensing. This reduces the chances of medication errors and improves documentation and inventory control.

pre-packing	Technicians often "pre-pack" medications that have been supplied in bulk into unit doses. Machines that automate this process are generally used for pre-packing oral solid medications.
medication order form	In the hospital, all drugs ordered for a patient are written on a medication order form and not a prescription blank as in a community pharmacy. Physicians write medication orders for hospital patients, though both nurses and pharmacists may also write orders if they are directly instructed to do so by a doctor. In addition, physician's assistants and nurse practitioners may sometimes write orders, depending upon the institution.
medication administration record	Nurses record and track medication orders on a patient specific form called the medication administration record (MAR).
controlled substances	A primary area of concern for inventory control is narcotics, or controlled substances, which require an exact record of the location of every item to the exact tablet or unit.
code carts	Locked carts filled with emergency medications. All patient care areas are required to have code carts.
IV admixtures	A large portion of the medication used in the hospital is administered intravenously. Pharmacy technicians prepare I.V. admixtures, including small and large volume parenterals, enteral nutrition therapy, and chemotherapy.
centralized pharmacy	A system in which all pharmacy activities are conducted from one location within the hospital: the inpatient pharmacy.
decentralized pharmacy	A system in which there are several pharmacy areas (called satellites) located throughout the hospital, each performing a specific function.
investigational drug service	A specialized pharmacy subsection that deals solely with clinical drug trials. These drug studies require a great deal of paperwork and special documentation of all doses of medication taken by patients. Technicians frequently assist the pharmacist with this documentation and in preparing individual patient medication supplies.
policy and procedures manual	A manual containing information about every aspect of the job from dress code to disciplinary actions and step by step directions on how to perform various tasks that will be required of technicians. All departments within the hospital are required by regulating agencies to maintain this.

KEY CONCEPTS

Test your knowledge by covering the information in the right hand column.

JCAHO	The Joint Commission on Accreditation of Healthcare Organizations, the accreditation agency for healthcare organizations. Organizations undergo a JCAHO survey every 3 years.
long-term care	Facilities that provide care for people unable to care for themselves because of mental or physical impairment. Because of limited resources, most long-term care facilities will contract out dispensing and clinical pharmacy services.
distributive pharmacist	A long-term care pharmacist responsible for making sure patients receive the correct medicines that were ordered.
consultant pharmacist	A long-term care pharmacist who develops and maintains an individualized pharmaceutical plan for every long-term care resident.
emergency kits	Locked kits containing emergency medications, similar to code carts used in hospitals.
automated dispensing stations	Automated units which dispense medications at the point of use.

unit dose medications

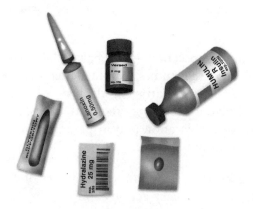

patient trays

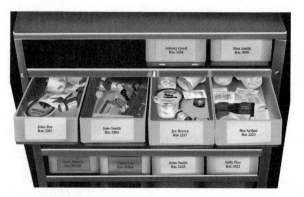

MEDICATION ORDERS

Medication order forms are an all-purpose communication tool used by the various members of the healthcare team. Orders for various procedures, laboratory tests, and x-rays may be written on the form in addition to medication orders. Several medication orders may be written on one medication order form unlike pharmacy prescription blanks seen in the retail setting.

There are several different types of orders that can be written. One is a standard medication order for patients to receive a certain drug at scheduled intervals throughout the day, sometimes called a standing order. Orders for medications that are administered only on an as needed basis are called PRN medication orders. A third type of order is for a medication that is needed right away and these are referred to as STAT orders.

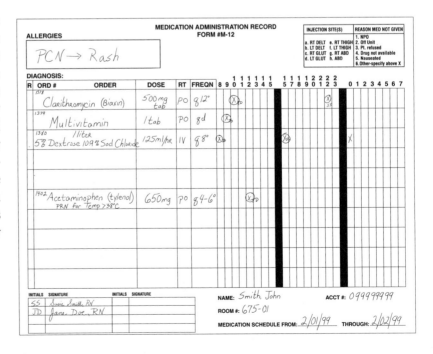

MEDICATION ADMINISTRATION RECORD

On this form every medication ordered for a patient is written down as well as the time it is administered and the person who gave the dose. These forms may be handwritten by the nursing staff or generated by the pharmacy computer system. The MAR is an important document in tracking the care of the patient as it gives a 24 hour picture of a patient's medication use. The accuracy of this document is crucial.

FILL IN THE KEY TERM

Answers are at the end of the book.

automated dispensing system
centralized pharmacy system
clean rooms
code carts
consultant pharmacist
decentralized pharmacy system
distributive pharmacist

inpatient pharmacy
Licensed Practical Nurse,
    L.P.N.
medication administration
    record (MAR)
Nurse Practitioner
outpatient pharmacy

policy and procedure manual
PRN order
Registered Nurse, R.N.
satellites
standing order
STAT order
unit dose

1. _____ : A registered nurse with additional training who can provide basic primary health care. The N.P. can prescribe various medications in most states.

2. _____ : A nurse who provides bedside care, assists physicians in various procedures, and administers medical regimens to patients.

3. _____ : A nurse who is not allowed to perform all functions of an R.N. and may not administer medication to patients.

4. _____ : A package containing the amount of a drug required for one dose.

5. _____ : A standard medication order for patients to receive medication at scheduled intervals.

6. _____ : An order for medication to be administered only on an as needed basis.

7. _____ : An order for medication to be administered immediately.

8. _____ : A form that tracks the medications administered to a patient.

9. _____ : A locked cart of medications designed for emergency use only.

10. _____ : A system in which all pharmacy activities in the hospital are conducted at one location, the inpatient pharmacy.

11. _____ : The hospital pharmacy in a centralized system.

12. _____ : A system in which pharmacy activities occur in multiple locations within a hospital.

13. _____ : Pharmacy locations in a decentralized systems that operate outside the central pharmacy.

14. _____ : Areas designed for the preparation of sterile products.

15. _____ : A pharmacy attached to a hospital servicing patients who have left the hospital or who are visiting doctors in a hospital outpatient clinic.

16. _____ : Documentation of required policies, procedures, and disciplinary actions in a hospital.

17. _____ : Makes sure long-term care patients receive the correct medications ordered.

18. _____ : Develops and maintains an individual pharmaceutical plan for each long-term care patient.

19. _____ : Automated unit which dispenses medications at the point of use.

TRUE/FALSE

Indicate whether the statement is true or false in the blank. Answers are at the end of the book.

_____ 1. An LPN supervises a Nurse Practitioner in the hospital setting.

_____ 2. Orders for medications that are needed immediately are PRN orders.

_____ 3. Technicians often prepare IV admixtures in hospitals.

_____ 4. Oral medications in hospitals are delivered to patient care areas in carts containing patient specific trays.

_____ 5. A centralized pharmacy system is made up of an inpatient pharmacy and satellite pharmacy areas.

_____ 6. All departments within a hospital are required to maintain a policy and procedure manual.

_____ 7. The consultant pharmacist develops and maintains an individual pharmaceutical plan for each long-term care patient.

EXPLAIN WHY

Explain why these statements are true or important. Check your answers in the text. Discuss any questions you may have with your Instructor.

1. Why can several medication orders be written on a single medication order form?

2. Why is it important for technicians to be familiar with the policy and procedures manual for their department?

— 17 —

OTHER ENVIRONMENTS

KEY CONCEPTS

Test your knowledge by covering the information in the right hand column.

mail order pharmacy	Delivery of prescriptions by mail (primarily for maintenance therapy). Mail order pharmacies are generally large scale operations that are highly automated. They use assembly line processing in which each step in the prescription fill process is completed or managed by a person who specializes in that step.
maintenance therapy	Therapy for chronic conditions that include depression, gastrointestinal disorders, heart disease, hypertension and diabetes.
regulation	Mail order pharmacies must follow federal and state requirements in processing prescriptions, but are not necessarily licensed in each state to which they send medications.
pharmacist review	Pharmacists review mail order prescriptions before and after filling.
home care	Care in the home, generally supervised by a registered nurse who works with a physician, pharmacist, and others to administer a care plan that involves the patient or another care giver.
home infusion	Infusion administered in the home, the fastest growing area of home health care. The primary therapies provided by home infusion services are: antibiotic therapy, parenteral nutrition, pain management and chemotherapy.
infusion pumps	Pumps that control infusion. There are pumps for specific therapies or multiple therapies, as well as ambulatory pumps that can be worn by patients.
patient education	In home infusion, the patient or their care giver is educated about their therapy: how to self-administer, monitor, report problems, and so on.
admixture preparation	The same rules apply to preparing parenteral admixtures in the home infusion setting as in the hospital.

TRUE/FALSE

Indicate whether the statement is true or false in the blank. Answers are at the end of the book.

_____ 1. A chronic condition is a serious condition that requires acute care therapy.

_____ 2. Mail order pharmacies are often used to handle maintenance medications.

_____ 3. Community pharmacy is growing more rapidly than mail order pharmacy.

_____ 4. Antibiotic therapy is a common home infusion service used in treating AIDS related and other infections.

_____ 5. On the home care team, the technician works under the supervision of a home care aide.

_____ 6. In home infusion, waste from chemotherapy and the treatment of AIDS patients can be safely disposed with the patient's other trash.

_____ 7. Pain management generally applies to the infusion of narcotics for patients with painful terminal illnesses or other types of severe chronic pain.

_____ 8. In home infusion, the stability of the admixture is a primary concern.

EXPLAIN WHY

Explain why these statements are true or important. Check your answers in the text. Discuss any questions you may have with your Instructor.

1. Why is mail order pharmacy growing so rapidly?

2. Why would maintenance drugs be well suited to mail order delivery?

3. Why is patient education important in home infusion?

4. Why is home infusion growing so rapidly?

5. Why is storage of admixtures an issue in home infusion?

6. Why is hazardous waste an issue in home infusion?

— Appendix A —

DRUG CLASSIFICATIONS

CLASSIFICATION OF DRUGS

There are thousands of drugs used in pharmacy. A basic familiarity with these drugs and their uses will enhance your skills as a pharmacy technician.

Drugs may be classified in different ways. One way is *based on their main therapeutic indication or action*. An example of such a group name would be **antibiotic**, which describes drugs that work by destroying pathogenic organisms (microorganisms that cause disease). Another example of a group name would be **analgesic**, which describes drugs that are used in the alleviation of pain. Following is a sample list of such group names:

Analgesics	Antitussives
Anesthetics	Antivirals
Antacids	Bronchodilators
Antibiotics	Cardiac Depressants
Anticoagulants	Decongestants
Anticonvulsants	Digestants
Antidiarrheals	Diuretics
Antiemetics	Hormones
Antihelmintics	Hypnotics
Antihistamines	Laxatives
Antineoplastics	Sedatives
Antiretrovirals	Tranquilizers

Another arrangement of drugs is by *specific classification based on how the drug actually works*. Drugs classified this way generally share these characteristics:

1. similar chemical structure
2. similar mechanism of action
3. similar effects (including side effects)

An example of such a classification is the **cephalosporins,** which is found in the antibiotics group. Drugs in the cephalosporins classification share the above mentioned characteristics with each other but not necessarily with other antibiotics, which may have different characteristics. Another example of such a group would be **xanthine derivatives**, which are found in the bronchodilators group.

Example:

Trade Name	Generic Name	Group	Classification
Keflex	Cephalexin	Antibiotic	Cephalosporin
Theo-Dur	Theophylline	Bronchodilator	Xanthine Derivative

Below is a sample list of such classifications:

Angiotensin Converting Enzyme inhibitors (ACE inhibitors)
α-adrenergic agonists
β-blockers
Calcium channel blockers
Cephalosporins
Corticosteroids
Histamine$_2$ blockers
Loop Diuretics

For the National Pharmacy Technician Certification Exam, you will need to know the main groups of drugs used in the retail and hospital setting. More specific classifications are not emphasized. You will learn most of this information on the job: as you handle these medications over and over again, you'll see which drugs are the most commonly used and which are not.

STUDY NOTES

Use this area to write important points you'd like to remember.

COMMON DRUGS

Pharmacy technicians should know drugs by both their trade name and generic name. It is also important to have a basic understanding of the drug's use. The following lists each of these elements for the most common drugs. Note that drugs often have different indications, and that we have only listed the indication that is the most common.

TRADE NAME	GENERIC NAME	MAIN INDICATION
Accupril	quinapril	antihypertensive
Adalet	nifedipine	antihypertensive
Advil	Ibuprofen	anti-inflammatory
Altase	ramipril	antihypertensive
Ambien	zolpidem	sedative / hypnotic
Amoxil	amoxicillin	antibiotic
Ativan	lorazepam	antianxiety
Atrovent	ipratropium	bronchodilator
Augmentin	amoxicillin / clavulanic acid	antibiotic
Axid	nizatidine	Inhibits stomach acid secretion
Azmacort	triamcinolone	bronchial asthma (inhaler)
Bactrim, Septra	sulfamethoxazole / trimethoprim	antibiotic
Bactroban	mupirocin	topical antibiotic
Beconase AQ	beclomethasone	bronchial asthma (inhaler)
Beepen-VK	penicillin V potassium	antibiotic
Biaxin	clarithromycin	antibiotic
Bumex	bumetanide	diuretic
BuSpar	buspirone	antianxiety
Calan SR	verapamil	antihypertensive
Capoten	captopril	antihypertensive
Carafate	sulcralfate	duodenal ulcer
Cardec DM	carbinoxamin, pseudoephedrine, and dextromethorphan	antihistamine / decongestant / antitussive
Cardizem CD	diltiazem	antihypertensive
Cardura	doxazosin	antihypertensive
Ceclor	cefaclor	antibiotic
Ceftin	cefuroxime	antibiotic
Cefzil	cefprozil	antibiotic
Cipro	ciprofloxacin	antibiotic
Claritin	loratidine	antihistamine
Compazine	prochlorperazine	antiemetics

TRADE NAME	GENERIC NAME	MAIN INDICATION
Contuss XT	guaifenesin and phenylpropanolamine	expectorant / decongestant
Coumadin	warfarin	anticoagulant
Cycrin	medroxyprogesterone	progestin
Darvocet-N	propoxyphene napsylate and acetaminophen	analgesic
Daypro	oxaprozin	anti-inflammatory
Deltasone	prednisone	anti-inflammatory
Demulen 1/35 28	ethinyl estradiol and ethynodial diacetate	oral contraceptive
Depakote	valproic acid	anticonvulsant
Desogen	ethinyl estradiol / desogestrel	oral contraceptive
Diflucan	fluconazole	antifungal
Dilantin	phenytoin	anticonvulsant
Duricef	cefadroxil	antibiotic
Dyazide	triamterene and hydrochlorothiazide	diuretic
DynaCirc	isradipine	antihypertensive
Elocon	mometasone	anti-inflammatory
Entex LA	guaifenesin and phenylpropanolamne	expectorant / decongestant
Erythrocin	erythromycin	antibiotic
Estrace	estradiol	estrogen
Estraderm	estradiol	estrogen (patch)
Fiorinal	butalbital / caffeine / aspirin	analgesic
Floxin	ofloxacin	antibiotic
Glucotrol	glipizide	antihyperglycemia (anti-diabetes)
DiaBeta	glyburide	antihyperglycemia (anti-diabetes)
Humulin	insulin (human)	antihyperglycemia (anti-diabetes)
Hytrin	terazosin	antihypertensive
Imitrex	sumaptriptan	for migraine
Intal	cromolyn sodium	bronchial asthma
K-Dur, Micro-K, Slow K	potassium chloride	potassium supplement
Keflex	cephalexin	antibiotic
Klonopin	clonazepam	antianxiety
Lanoxin	digoxin	increase cardiac output
Lasix	furosemide	diuretic
Levoxyl	levothyroxine	anti-hypothyroidism

TRADE NAME	GENERIC NAME	MAIN INDICATION
Lo/Ovral 28	ethinyl estradiol / norgestrel	oral contraceptive
Lodine	etodolac	anti-inflammatory
Loestrin-FE 1.5/30	ethinyl estradiol / norethindrone	oral contraceptive
Lopressor	metoprolol	antihypertensive
Lorabid	loracarbef	antibiotic
Lorcet Plus	hydrocodone / acetaminophen	analgesic
Lotrisone	betamethasone dipropionate and clotrimazole	anti-inflammatory /antifungal (topical)
Lozol	indapamide	diuretic
Macrobid	nitrofurantoin	antibiotic
Mevacor	lovastatin	antihyperlipidemia
Naprosyn	naproxen	anti-inflammatory
Nasacort	triamcinolone	anti-inflammatory (nasal inhaler)
Nitrostat, Nitro-Dur	nitroglycerin	antianginal
Nizoral	ketoconazole	antifungal
Nolvadex	tamoxifen	anti-estrogen
Norvasc	amlodipine	antihypertensive
Ogen	estropipate	estrogen
Ortho-Cept 28	ethinyl estradiol and desogestrel	oral contraceptive
Ortho-Novum 7/7/7-28	ethinyl estradiol and norethindrone	oral contraceptive
Oruvail	ketoprofen	anti-inflammatory
Paxil	paroxetine	antidepressant
Penicillin VK, Pen Vee K, Veetids	penicillin V potassium	antibiotic
Pepcid	famotidine	inhibits stomach acid secretion
Percocet	oxycodone / acetaminophen	analgesic
Peridex	chlorhexidine	gingivitis
Phenergan	promethazine	antiemetics
Pravachol	pravastatin	antihyperlipidemia
Premarin	conjugated estrogen	estrogen
Prilosec	omeprazole	inhibits stomach acid secretion
Principen	ampicillin	antibiotic
Prinivil	lisinopril	antihypertensive
Procardia	nifedipine	antihypertensive
Propacet	propoxyphene / acetaminophen	analgesic
Propulsid	cisapride	gastrointestinal stimulant

TRADE NAME	GENERIC NAME	MAIN INDICATION
Proventil, Ventolin	albuterol	bronchodilator
Provera	medroxyprogesterone	progestin
Prozac	fluoxetine	antidepressant
Relafen	nabumetone	anti-inflammatory
Retin-A	tretinoin	anti acne (topical)
Ritalin	methylphenidate	attention deficit disorder (ADD)
Slo-Bid, Theo-Dur	theophylline	bronchodilator
Sumycin	tetracycline	antibiotic
Suprax	cefixime	antibiotic
Synthroid	levothyroxine	anti-hypothyroidism
Tagamet	cimetidine	inhibits stomach acid secretion
Tegretol	carbamazepine	anticonvulsant
Tenormin	atenolol	antihypertensive
Terazol	terconazole	antifungal
Timoptic	timolol	glaucoma (eye)
Tobradex	tobramycin / dexamethasone	antibiotic / anti-inflammatory (eye)
Toradol	ketorolac	anti-inflammatory / analgesic
Trental	pentoxifylline	enhance circulation
Tri-Levlen-28, Triphasil	ethinyl estradiol levonorgestrel	oral contraceptive
Tussionex	hydrocodone and chlorpheniramine	antitussive / antihistamine
Tylenol with codeine	acetaminophen / codeine	analgesic
Valium	diazepam	antianxiety
Vancenase AQ Vanceril	beclomethasone	bronchial asthma (inhaler)
Vantin	cefpodoxime	antibiotic
Vasotec	enalapril	antihypertensive
Vicodin	hydrocodone / acetaminophen	analgesic
Voltaren	diclofenac	anti-inflammatory
Xanax	alprazolam	antianxiety
Zantac	ranitidine	inhibits stomach acid secretion
Zestril	lisinopril	antihypertensive
Zithromax	azithromycin	antibiotic
Zocor	simvastatin	antihyperlipidemia
Zoloft	sertraline	antidepressant
Zovirax	acyclovir	antiviral

KEY CONCEPTS

Test your knowledge by covering the information in the right hand column.

USAN

The United States Adopted Names Council (USAN) designates nonproprietary names for drugs.

drug classes

Group names for drugs that have similar activities or are used for the same type of diseases and disorders.

stems

Common stems or syllables that are used to identify the different drug classes and in making new nonproprietary names. They are approved and recommended by the USAN.

neurotransmitter

Chemicals released by nerves that interact with receptors to cause an effect.

homeostasis

The state of equilibrium of the body.

epilepsy

A chronic disorder characterized by recurring seizures with symptoms such as fainting and muscle spasms.

anticonvulsants

Drugs that reduce epileptic seizure frequency. The primary anticonvulsant drugs are: phenytoin, carbamazepine, valproic acid. Nearly all anticonvulsants can cause side effects ranging from minor to severe, including drug-induced seizures if blood concentrations are too high.

diabetes

A common disorder caused by a deficiency of the hormone insulin or an inability of the body to use it effectively. Diabetic symptoms include abnormally high levels of blood glucose, increased urination, thirst, and weight loss. Insulin administration is the principal treatment for diabetes mellitus, but is not a cure. Diabetic patients are prone to heart disease, circulatory problems, eye disorders, and infections of the feet.

antiemetics

Emesis (vomiting) is a common adverse effect of chemotherapy given to cancer patients. Centrally acting dopamine antagonists and serotonin receptor antagonists are used.

gout

A disorder in uric acid excretion that is characterized by hyperuricemia, an abnormal concentration of uric acid in the blood.

antihyperlipidemics

Hyperlipidemia is known to cause atherosclerosis (a narrowing of the arteries), a major risk factor in heart attack and stroke. Antihyperlipidemics lower cholesterol and triglyceride levels. They include the "-vastatin" (or "-statin") drugs that block the body's synthesis of cholesterol.

hypertension (HTN)

Abnormally high blood pressure, a major risk factor for heart disease, diabetes, and other serious conditions. Blood pressure is written (in mm Hg) as a relationship of systolic to diastolic pressures (e.g, 120/80). Normal pressure ranges differ according to gender and age. A systolic pressure of 120-140

hypertension (cont'd)	and a diastolic pressure of 80-89 are normal for most adults, though this does vary somewhat by individual. Men have higher pressures than women, and older people have higher pressures than younger people. Beta-blockers (β-blockers) lower blood pressure by lowering cardiac output. Calcium channel blockers lower blood pressure by relaxing blood vessels.
antibiotic	Drugs that suppress the growth of other microorganisms. Antimicrobial refers to both synthetic agents and natural antibiotics. Penicillins and cephalosporins are the major classes of antibiotics that work by inhibiting cell wall synthesis in bacteria. Aminoglycosides, macrolides, and tetracyclines act by interfering with the microorganism's ability to synthesize proteins. Erythromycin, the first and still most widely used macrolide antibiotic, has been used since 1952. Tetracyclines are mainly bacteriostatic, but at high concentrations, can be bactericidal. Sulfonamides, the first bacterial agents, are antibiotics that interfere with folic acid synthesis. They should be taken with plenty of water. The quinolones inhibit an enzyme involved with DNA replication. A major drug interaction can occur between the quinolones and such cations as zinc and calcium.
bactericidal	Kills bacteria.
bacteriostatic	Retards bacteria growth.
antimycobacterial agents	Drugs that kill mycobacteria, microorganisms that cause tuberculosis, leprosy, and Mycobacterium avium complex (MAC) disease in AIDS patients.
tuberculosis	An infectious disease which primarily affects the respiratory system. The primary antituberculosis drugs include isoniazid, pyrazinamide, ethambutol, ethionamide, and rifampin. Therapy generally involves a combination of drugs.
leprosy	The primary drug used to treat leprosy is dapsone, which is chemically similar to the sulfonamides. The controversial drug thalidomide has received new use in treating leprosy.
antifungals	Miconazole was marketed in 1974 as the first azole-type antifungal agent. The "-azoles" work by changing the fungus cell membrane to cause it contents to leak out.
anti-protozoal agents	Protozoa are single cell organisms that have infected humans for thousands of years. Many different drugs having different mechanisms of action are used to treat protozoal infections.
antimalarials	Malaria has been one of the most fatal diseases in human history from ancient times to the present. The quinoline derivatives are still the most important antimalarial agents.

KEY CONCEPTS

Test your knowledge by covering the information in the right hand column.

antihelminthic agents	Worms cause "helminthic" infections. Drug therapy is based on the infecting organism.
urinary tract infections (UTIs)	Treated with antiseptics and anti-infectives that inhibit bacterial growth in the urinary tract.
cancer	Cancer cells disregard the normal controls on cellular growth. They multiply out of control, have abnormal genetic content, and are generally non-functional. Tumors (also called neoplasms or cancers), are either benign (non-progressive) or malignant (spreading, growing worse).
antineoplastics	Chemotherapy involves using multiple drugs that act on cancer cells in different ways and have multiple side effects. It's given in cycles, with rest periods that allow the patient to recover. Alkylating agents interfere with cell metabolism and growth. Antimetabolites prevent cancer cell growth by affecting its DNA. Hormonal antineoplastics either block hormone production or hormone action.
Parkinson's Disease	A progressive disorder of the nervous system characterized by muscle tremors, weakness, and rigidity or stiffness of joints. Parkinson's disease is associated with reduced dopamine levels in the brain, and Anti-Parkinson drugs are designed to increase dopamine levels.
antivirals	Viruses invade host cells and use the DNA or RNA of the host cell to copy or replicate themselves. They cannot replicate themselves independently. Some antivirals act by blocking steps in the viral replication process.
corticosteroids	Cortisol (also called hydrocortisone) is produced in the adrenal glands and is the primary corticosteroid in humans. Cortisol produces a wide range of effects that influence metabolism, modify the response of the immune system, and produce anti-inflammatory activity. Corticosteroids are absorbed through the skin and into the vascular system, so careful application is needed to avoid systemic effects.
dermatologicals	Many different conditions or diseases are localized on or in the skin, requiring many different classes of drugs to be used in treatment. Conditions or diseases of the skin range from dermatitis caused by irritants or allergens to viral infections to severe burns. Product formulations used as dermatologicals also vary widely: ointments, creams, lotions, shampoos, sprays, bath additives, tapes, etc.

stomach acid agents

Secretion of stomach acid is regulated by histamine, acetylcholine, and other intestinal enzymes. Antacids neutralize existing stomach acid. Sucralfate is an aluminum salt that acts with proteins at the ulcer site to form a protective layer. H_2-receptor antagonists block the effects of histamine in stimulating gastric acid. The first H_2-receptor antagonist was cimetidine and overnight, antacid therapy became outmoded. The brand drug, Tagamet® is probably one of the most prescribed drugs of all time.

antidiarrheals

Antiperistaltic drugs treat diarrhea by inhibiting the movements (peristalsis) of the intestine. Adsorbent drugs work by attaching bacteria, toxins, and nutrients to their surface. Antibiotics have both positive and negative effects in treating diarrhea. Some antibiotics kill the naturally occurring bacterial flora of the intestinal tract, and this can lead to diarrhea.

laxatives and stool softeners

The colon plays a significant role in fluid balance and excretion. Constipation occurs when fecal material in the colon becomes dehydrated. Laxatives should not be used chronically as they may cause dependence.

nitrates

Nitrates are vasodilators, drugs that relax and expand the blood vessels. They reduce the heart's workload by reducing the amount of blood supplied to it. This reduces the pressure on the heart. The first nitrate, nitroglycerin, is still considered the drug of choice.

beta blockers (β-blockers)

When these drugs are used to treat angina, they produce a reduction in myocardial oxygen demand and a reduction in the number of anginal attacks. Another benefit of these drugs is that they limit the severity and recurrence of myocardial infarctions (heart attacks). The β-blockers have many non-cardiovascular applications. They are used to reduce essential tremor, prevent anxiety, treat migraine headaches, and treat glaucoma. The first β-blocker was propranolol.

calcium channel blockers

Relax the heart by reducing conduction and contraction. They also help the heart by relaxing the blood vessels.

antiarrhythmics

Disturbances in the rate or rhythm of the heartbeat are called arrhythmias. Arrhythmias may cause too rapid (tachycardia), too slow (bradycardia), or unsynchronized heart muscle contractions (premature contractions) and result in a decrease in the volume of blood pumped by the heart. There are different classes of antiarrhythmic drugs based on their specific effects and mechanisms of action.

isomer

A variation of a drug that has the same molecular formula but a different arrangement of the atoms in the molecule.

KEY CONCEPTS

Test your knowledge by covering the information in the right hand column.

inotropes	Drugs that increase the force of cardiac contraction. There are three classes: digitalis glycosides, adrenergic receptor agonists, and phosphodiesterase inhibitors. Dopamine and dobutamine are used as inotropes.
coagulation enhancers	Blood coagulation involves a complex interaction of platelets, proteins, and tissue materials. Clotting factors exist in the blood in inactive form and must be converted to an active form before clotting can be accomplished. Many coagulation enhancers have been produced from human plasma.
anemia	A deficiency of red blood cells, a common side effect of chemotherapy.
hematopoietic drugs	Assist or stimulate the growth of blood cells.
anticoagulants	Act against blood clot formation. Abnormal blood clot formation within blood vessels can cause heart attack, stroke, or pulmonary embolism (a blood clot in the lung).
hemostatic drugs	Prevent excessive bleeding. Systemic hemostatic agents include aminocaproic acid, tranexamic acid, and aprotinin.
thyroid hormones	Involved in many of the body's essential processes, including growth, metabolism, and CNS development. Hypothyroidism is treated by the administration of thyroid hormone. The treatment of hyperthyroidism is more complex. Anti-thyroid drugs, radioactive iodine, or surgery are used to reduce the effects of the excess hormone. Anti-thyroid drugs block the synthesis of the thyroid hormones.
oral contraceptives	The female sex hormones estrogens and the progestins control the development of female secondary sex characteristics, the menstrual cycle, ovulation, pregnancy, and many metabolic processes. Since their release, amounts of estrogen and progestin in oral contraceptives have been greatly reduced, resulting in fewer side effects. Oral contraceptives now contain ethinyl estradiol or mestranol as the estrogen component and norethindrone, norgestrel, or ethynodiol diacetate as the progestin component.
ovulation stimulants	The so-called "fertility agents" used to stimulate or assist the ovulation process in infertility. Human chorionic gonadotropin (HCG) was the first agent used to treat infertility. Multiple births are common when using these fertility agents.
oxytocic and tocolytic agents	Oxytocic agents stimulate uterine contractions. Tocolytic agents cause uterine relaxation. Stimulation of the uterus is used in abortion, induction of labor, or postpartum hemorrhage.

oxytocic and tocolytic agents (cont'd)	Uterine relaxants are used to prevent or arrest preterm labor, reverse stimulation by oxytocic agents, facilitate uterine manipulations, and relieve painful contractions during menstruation.
androgens	The pharmacological activity of androgens is the basis of male sex characteristics. It is responsible for the normal growth and development of the male sex organs and secondary sex characteristics such as hair distribution, vocal cord thickening, body musculature and fat distribution. Testosterone, the most important androgen in males, is produced in the testis.
finasteride	Finasteride (Proscar®) is a synthetic steroid that is used to reduce the size of the prostate in benign prostatic hyperplasia (BPH). Finasteride (Propecia®), the same drug but in a different dosage form, is indicated for male pattern baldness. Finasteride may cause abnormalities in a male fetus, and women who are or may become pregnant should not be exposed to this drug in any form.
anabolic steroids	Anabolic steroids are derived from or are closely related to the androgen testosterone. They promote the body tissue building processes and reverse the tissue depleting processes. Because of the potential for abuse, the anabolic steroids are scheduled as C-III controlled substances.
immunoglobulins	One of the primary components of the immune system, they provide immunization to one or more infectious diseases. They are obtained from donor plasma.
monoclonal antibodies	Genetically engineered monoclonal antibodies are immunoglobulins that have the advantage of being able to be produced in an unlimited supply.
immunosuppressive agents	Used in transplant surgery to prevent organ rejection.
neuromuscular blockers	Relax muscles or produce muscle paralysis. They are often used as adjuncts (not replacements) to anesthesia during surgery.
skeletal muscle relaxants	Drugs with sedative properties that generally reduce pain rather than directly relaxing muscles.
antiglaucoma drugs	Drugs that lower the pressure in the eye that is caused by glaucoma.
mydriatics	Drugs that dilate the pupil, often for eye examinations.
allergic conjunctivitis	Inflammation of the conjunctiva caused by allergy. Drugs that block the release of histamine are used to treat it.
artificial tears	Lubricating solutions that are isotonic, buffered, and pH adjusted and stay in contact with the eye for prolonged periods.

KEY CONCEPTS

Test your knowledge by covering the information in the right hand column.

analgesic drugs	Drugs that block or reduce the perception of pain but not its cause. Analgesics fall into three groups. Two groups of drugs are used for mild to moderate pain. They are the nonsteroidal anti-inflammatory drugs (NSAIDs) and the salicylates (aspirin being the best known example). Some of these drugs also have antipyretic (fever reducing) activity and anti-inflammatory activity. NSAIDs vary greatly between patients in their effectiveness. The third group, the opioids, is used in cases of more severe pain. This class of drugs is also called "narcotic analgesics" and have a very high abuse potential.
Reye's Syndrome	A potentially fatal disorder associated with the use of aspirin in treating children with viral infections.
local anesthetics	Local anesthetics are used to decrease pain, temperature, touch sensation, and skeletal muscle tone. Cocaine was the first local anesthetic. In 1905, the first synthetic local anesthetic, procaine, was made. The more common local anesthetics today are lidocaine, bupivacaine, and tetracaine.
general anesthesia	A condition with these four characteristics: unconsciousness, analgesia, muscle relaxation, and reflex depression. A combination of anesthetics that can include both inhaled and intravenous agents are used in general anesthesia to produce a balanced anesthetic effect. This is because different anesthetics have different effects.
psychotropic agents	Drugs that affect behavior, psychotic state, and sleep. They are used to treat schizophrenia, depression, mania, anxiety, and arousal, and are grouped into three categories: antidepressants, antipsychotics (major tranquilizers), and sedatives-hypnotics.
antidepressants	Drugs used to treat depression. Monoamine oxidase inhibitors (MAOIs) have a potentially severe drug-diet interaction with aged cheeses, sausages, and red wine. Tricyclic antidepressants have side effects that include dry mouth, blurred vision, constipation, sedation, and sexual dysfunction. Selective Serotonin Reuptake Inhibitors (SSRIs) are antidepressants for which the primary side effect is nausea.
antipsychotics	Also called tranquilizers or neuroleptics, they decrease conditioned behavioral responses, cause a lack of initiative and interest, blunt emotions, and produce limited sedation. They have various side effects, depending upon their action. These include rapid heart beat, difficulty urinating, memory impairment, and muscle spasms.

sedatives

Sedatives reduce anxiety or produce a calming effect. The benzodiazepines, introduced in the 1960s, are the primary anxiolytic drugs.

hypnotics

Hypnotic drugs are used to produce sleep or drowsiness.

asthma

Asthma is characterized by the obstruction of the pulmonary airways. The lungs of asthma patients are hypersensitive to common allergens. Treatment of asthma generally involves a multi-step strategy. Such an approach might include: avoidance of the causing factors when possible; use of cromolyn and nedocromil to prevent histamine release; use of anti-inflammatory drugs which include corticosteroids; use of drugs that can reverse bronchoconstriction or inhibit its development; use of drugs that reduce the frequency of recurrent attacks of bronchospasm; use of bronchodilators. Inhaled corticosteroids are a common treatment for asthma. Metered dose inhalers are generally used to deliver measured doses.

antihistamines

Antihistamines are H_1-receptor antagonists. Many antihistamines also antagonize various other receptors, which accounts for the number of additional effects seen with the antihistamines. These include dryness of the mouth, antipruritic (anti-itch), sedative, antiemetic, anti-motion sickness, antiparkinsonian, antitussive, and local anesthetic properties.

decongestants

Drugs that increase drainage and reduce congestion by shrinking mucous membranes.

antitussive

A drug that acts against a cough. They can be divided into two groups: narcotics and non-narcotics. The narcotics codeine and hydrocodone have antitussive properties when used at a lower dose than required to produce analgesia. Non-narcotic antitussives decrease the cough reflex without inducing many of the common characteristics of narcotic preparations. Dextromethorphan, diphenhydramine, and benzonatate are members of this class.

expectorants

Guaifenesin is the only expectorant recognized as safe and effective by the FDA.

shock

Shock occurs when there is not enough blood flow to deliver the necessary oxygen and nutrients to cells and tissues. This interferes with normal cell function, and if severe enough, can result in death. The treatment of shock begins with the administration of fluids. Vasopressors are used to increase blood pressure and stimulate circulation.

FILL IN THE BLANKS

Match the brand name with the generic and the indictation. Answers are at the end of the book.

Advil	Carafate	Erythrocin	Nolvadex	Ritalin
Amoxil	Cardizem CD	Fiorinal	Pepcid	Tagamet
Ativan	Ceclor	Humulin	Percocet	Tenormin
Augmentin	Ceftin	Imitrex	Pravachol	Valium
Axid	Claritin	Keflex	Prilosec	Vancenase AQ
Bactrim	Cycrin	Lanoxin	Procardia	Vicodin
Bactroban	Daypro	Lasix	Proventil	Voltaren
Biaxin	Deltasone	Lo/Ovral 28	Prozac	Zantac
BuSpar	Desogen	Mevacor	Relafen	Zithromax
Capoten	Dilantin	Naprosyn	Retin-A	Zocor

1. _____ : albuterol — bronchodilator

2. _____ : amoxicillin — antibiotic

3. _____ : amoxicillin / clavulanic acid — antibiotic

4. _____ : atenolol — antihypertensive

5. _____ : azithromycin — antibiotic

6. _____ : beclomethasone — bronchial asthma (inhaler)

7. _____ : buspirone — antianxiety

8. _____ : butalbital / caffeine / aspirin — analgesic

9. _____ : captopril — antihypertensive

10. _____ : sucralfate — duodenal ulcer

11. _____ : cefaclor — antibiotic

12. _____ : cefuroxime — antibiotic

13. _____ : cephalexin — antibiotic

14. _____ : cimetidine — inhibits stomach acid secretion

15. _____ : clarithromycin — antibiotic

16. _____ : sulfamethoxazole / trimethoprim — antibiotic

17. _____ : diazepam — antianxiety

18. _____ : diclofenac — anti-inflammatory

19. _____ : digoxin — increase cardiac output

20. _____ : diltiazem — antihypertensive

21. _____ : erythromycin — antibiotic

22. _____	:	ethinyl estradiol / desogestrel	oral contraceptive
23. _____	:	ethinyl estradiol / norgestrel	oral contraceptive
24. _____	:	famotidine	inhibits stomach acid secretion
25. _____	:	fluoxetine	antidepressant
26. _____	:	furosemide	diuretic
27. _____	:	hydrocodone / acetaminophen	analgesic
28. _____	:	ibuprofen	anti-inflammatory
29. _____	:	insulin (human)	antihyperglycemia (anti-diabetes)
30. _____	:	loratidine	antihistamine
31. _____	:	lorazepam	antianxiety
32. _____	:	lovastatin	antihyperlipidemia
33. _____	:	medroxyprogesterone	progestin
34. _____	:	methylphenidate	attention deficit disorder (ADD)
35. _____	:	mupirocin	topical antibiotic
36. _____	:	nabumetone	anti-inflammatory
37. _____	:	naproxen	anti-inflammatory
38. _____	:	nifedipine	antihypertensive
39. _____	:	nizatidine	inhibits stomach acid secretion
40. _____	:	omeprazole	inhibits stomach acid secretion
41. _____	:	oxaprozin	anti-inflammatory
42. _____	:	oxycodone / acetaminophen	analgesic
43. _____	:	phenytoin	anticonvulsant
44. _____	:	pravastatin	antihyperlipidemia
45. _____	:	prednisone	anti-inflammatory
46. _____	:	ranitidine	inhibits stomach acid secretion
47. _____	:	simvastatin	antihyperlipidemia
48. _____	:	sumaptriptan	for migraine
49. _____	:	tamoxifen	anti-estrogen
50. _____	:	tretinoin	anti acne (topical)

FILL IN THE KEY TERM

Answers are at the end of the book.

anabolic steroids	bactericidal	decongestants	monoclonal antibodies
analgesic drugs	bacteriostatic	expectorants	mydriatics
anemia	beta blockers	gout	neuromuscular blockers
anticoagulants	calcium channel	hematopoietic drugs	nitrates
antiemetics	blockers	immunoglobulins	Parkinson's disease
antihyperlipidemics	chemotherapy	inotropes	sedatives
antipsychotics	cimetidine	insulin	tuberculosis
antitussive	dapsone	isomer	

1. _____ : The principal treatment for diabetes mellitus, but not a cure.

2. _____ : Often given to patients receiving chemotherapy to prevent vomiting.

3. _____ : A disorder in uric acid excretion that is characterized by hyperuricemia, an abnormal concentration of uric acid in the blood.

4. _____ : Drugs that lower cholesterol and triglyceride levels.

5. _____ : Kills bacteria.

6. _____ : Retards bacteria growth.

7. _____ : An infectious disease which primarily affects the respiratory system.

8. _____ : The primary drug used to treat leprosy.

9. _____ : Multiple drug therapy that acts on cancer cells in different ways and have multiple side effects.

10. _____ : A progressive disorder of the nervous system characterized by muscle tremors, weakness, and rigidity or stiffness of joints.

11. _____ : An H_2-receptor antagonist that blocks the effects of histamine in stimulating gastric acid. The brand name drug is Tagamet®.

12. _____ : Vasodilators that reduce the heart's workload by reducing the amount of blood supplied to it.

13. _____ : Drugs used to treat angina, lower blood pressure, and for many non-cardiovascular applications. The first one was propanolol.

14. _____ : Drugs that relax the heart and blood vessels.

15. _____ : A variation of a drug that has the same molecular formula but a different arrangement of the atoms in the molecule.

16. _____ : Drugs that increase the force of cardiac contraction.

17. _____ : A deficiency of red blood cells, a common side effect of chemotherapy.

18. _____ : Assist or stimulate the growth of blood cells.

19. _____ : Act against blood clot formation.

20. _____ : Promote the body tissue building processes and reverse the tissue depleting processes.

21. _____ : One of the primary components of the immune system, they provide immunization to one or more infectious diseases.

22. _____ : Genetically engineered immunoglobulins.

23. _____ : Relax muscles or produce muscle paralysis.

24. _____ : Drugs that dilate the pupil, often for eye examinations.

25. _____ : Drugs that block or reduce the perception of pain but not its cause.

26. _____ : Also called tranquilizers or neuroleptics.

27. _____ : Drugs that reduce anxiety or produce a calming effect.

28. _____ : Drugs that increase drainage and reduce congestion by shrinking mucous membranes.

29. _____ : A drug that acts against a cough.

30. _____ : Guaifenesin is the only drug in this classification recognized as safe and effective by the FDA.

STUDY TIP — DRUG CARDS

A good way to help you remember the most common drugs used in pharmacy is to create drug cards. Drug cards are easy to make by writing the information from the previous list on small index cards. You can then use these to study until you have memorized the information.

Information needed on your drug card:

1. Trade name of drug

2. Generic name of drug

3. Main indication
   Note: Many drugs have more than one indication. You need to know only the main indication.

PRACTICE EXAM

The following multiple choice questions are in the *choose the best answer format* of the National Pharmacy Technician Certification Examination. There are four possible answers with only one answer being the most correct. Many of these questions can be answered through a careful review of this workbook. However, others require knowledge gained from practice as a technician. Answers for all questions can be found at the end of the exam.

Since the time limit for taking the National Exam is three hours, you may want to test your ability to answer the questions under a time limit, or you may simply wish to time yourself to see how long it takes you. There are 125 questions here, the same number as on the exam. If you wish to have a similar experience, you can allow yourself three hours to answer these questions.

For more information on the National Exam, see the preface of this Workbook.

Answers are at the end of the exam.

1. The cost of 120 grams of triamcinolone 0.1% cream is $45.00. What would be the cost of 15 grams?

    a. $2.42
    b. $5.63
    c. $8.45
    d. $10.45

2. The approximate metric weight of sixteen ounces is

    a. 240 grams
    b. 254 grams
    c. 500 grams
    d. 454 grams

3. Opiates or narcotics are generally found in this classification.

    a. Schedule II
    b. Schedule III
    c. Schedule IV
    d. Schedule V

4. Most drugs are metabolized by the

    a. liver
    b. kidneys
    c. gall bladder
    d. gastrointestinal tract

5. Nolvadex® or _____ is an anti-estrogen type medication that is often used in the treatment of breast cancer.

    a. albuterol
    b. tamoxifen
    c. phenytoin
    d. nifedipine

6. Tylenol No. 3 is acetaminophen 325 mg and codeine _____mg.

    a. 15 mg
    b. 30 mg
    c. 60 mg
    d. none of the above

Answers are at the end of the exam.

7.   When using a Class A torsion balance,

   a.   the weight goes on the left pan and the powder goes on the right pan.
   b.   the weight goes on the right pan and the powder goes on the left pan.
   c.   Class A torsion balance only has one pan in which the powder goes.
   d.   can weigh amounts smaller than 120 milligrams

8.   The form number for ordering Schedule II drugs is:

   a.   DEA Form 121
   b.   DEA Form 200
   c.   DEA Form 222
   d.   DEA Form 240

9.   Which drug can be used as a patch?

   a.   nupercainal ointment
   b.   clonidine
   c.   amoxicillin
   d.   vitamin C

10.   How much diluent do you need to add to a 4 gm vial to get a concentration of 250 mg / ml. Disregard the space the powder may occupy.

   a.   12 ml
   b.   14 ml
   c.   16 ml
   d.   18 ml

11.   The smallest gelatin capsule used for extemporaneous compounding is size

   a.   10
   b.   8
   c.   5
   d.   000

12.   Which type of drug would be considered a drug of abuse?

   a.   opiates
   b.   alcohol
   c.   nicotine
   d.   all of the above

Answers are at the end of the exam.

13. Furosemide or Lasix® is used as

    a. an analgesic
    b. an anti-inflammatory agent
    c. a sedative
    d. a diuretic

14. The infusion rate of an IV is over 12 hours. The total exact volume is 800 ml. What would be the infusion rate in mls per minute?

    a. 0.56 ml / minute
    b. 1.11 ml / minute
    c. 2.7 ml / minute
    d. none of the above

15. You have a 70% solution of dextrose. How many grams of dextrose is in 400 ml of this solution?

    a. 700 grams
    b. 460 grams
    c. 280 grams
    d. 120 grams

16. The standard pediatric dose for cefazolin is 20 mg/kg/day. The order is written for 150 mg TID. The infant weighs 8 lb. Is this dose:

    a. too high
    b. too low
    c. within guidelines

17. Factors affecting oral route of administration would include:

    a. age
    b. body weight
    c. time of administration
    d. all of the above

18. An IV order calls for the addition of 45 mEq of $CaCO_3$ (calcium carbonate). You have a 25 ml vial of $CaCO_3$ 4.4mEq/ml. How many mls of this concentrate do you need to add to this IV?

    a. 5.6 ml
    b. 8.4 ml
    c. 10.2 ml
    d. 12.8 ml

Answers are at the end of the exam.

19. In this formula, how much talc is needed to fill 120 grams?

    nupercainal ointment   4%
    zinc oxide   20%
    talc 2%

    a. 2400 mg
    b. 1500 mg
    c. 2000 mg
    d. 2400 mg

20. A bottle of nitroglycerin has the labeled strength of 1/200 grains. What would this strength be in milligrams?

    a. 0.2 mg
    b. 0.3 mg
    c. 0.4 mg
    d. 0.6 mg

21. A pharmacy wants to mark-up a product by thirty percent. How much would an item cost with this mark-up, if its original cost was $4.50?

    a. $5.85
    b. $6.23
    c. $6.40
    d. $7.10

22. Until recently, all of the anticonvulsant drugs have been used for decades. Which one of the following drugs is a new drug in the arsenal of anticonvulsant therapy?

    a. phenobarbital
    b. diazepam
    c. phenytoin
    d. gabapentin

23. The Material Safety Data Sheets (MSDS)

    a. provide protocols for fire hazards in the pharmacy setting
    b. provide safety codes by OSHA in the storage of inventory
    c. provide information concerning hazardous substances
    d. none of the above

Answers are at the end of the exam.

24. How much diluent do you need to add to 4 gm of a powder to get a concentration of 250 mg/ml?

   a. 12 ml
   b. 16 ml
   c. 20 ml
   d. none of the above

25. What does DAW mean on a written prescription?

   a. the medication ordered is a controlled substance
   b. the medication should be taken with water
   c. the brand name is to be dispensed as written
   d. refills are limited to six months

26. This reference book contains official drug standards and is a required reference source in all licensed pharmacy settings.

   a. USP
   b. Facts & Comparisons
   c. Martindales
   d. American Drug Index

27. The last set of digits of the NDC are indicative of

   a. the manufacturer
   b. product identification
   c. package size
   d. none of the above

28. The approximate size container for the dispensing of 180 ml of liquid medication would be?

   a.) 2 ounces
   b.) 4 ounces
   c.) 6 ounces
   d.) 8 ounces

29. A patient asks whether he/she can take a certain medication with another one? As a pharmacy technician what should you do?

   a. inform the patient that you see no problem
   b. provide the patient with a drug insert
   c. request the patient see the pharmacist for a consult
   d. try to sell the patient some Mylanta®

127

Answers are at the end of the exam.

30. The doctor writes: ii gtts OU bid. What does this mean?

    a. two drops in the left eye twice a day
    b. two drops in the right eye twice a day
    c. two drops in each eye twice a day
    d. two drops in the right ear twice a day

31. Which of the following suppositories should be stored in the refrigerator?

    a. Phenergan®
    b. Thorazine®
    c. Tigan®
    d. Compazine®

32. Which of the following books is used for FDAs list of approved drug products?

    a. Merck Index
    b. Red Book
    c. Orange Book
    d. Martindale

33. Propranolol is the same as

    a. inderal
    b. tenormin
    c. lisinopril
    d. propulsid

34. Thiazide diuretics are used to:

    a. relieve migraine headaches
    b. relieve gastroenteritis
    c. manage of pain
    d. manage the retention of water

35. Of the following, which one deals with the issue of safety caps on prescription bottles?

    a. The Controlled Substance Act
    b. The Poison Prevention Act
    c. Hazardous Substance Act
    d. Federal Food and Cosmetic Act

Answers are at the end of the exam.

36. An example of a major drug-drug interaction would be:

    a. warfarin-aspirin
    b. digoxin-diltiazem
    c. penicillin-cephalosporin
    d. hydrocodone-codeine

37. The appearance of crystals in mannitol injection would indicate that the product:

    a. was exposed to cold
    b. has settled during shipment
    c. contains impurities and should be returned
    d. was formulated using sterile saline

38. How many 30 mg $KMNO_4$ (Potassium Permanganate) tablets are needed to make the following solution: $KMNO_4$ 1:5000 600 ml

    a. 2 tablets
    b. 3 tablets
    c. 4 tablets
    d. 6 tablets

39. Dextrose 25% 1000ml is ordered. You have only dextrose 70% solution available. How much of the dextrose 70% solution and sterile water will you use to fill this order?

    a. 250 ml dextrose 70% and 750 ml sterile water
    b. 357 ml dextrose 70% and 643 ml sterile water
    c. 424 ml dextrose 70% and 576 ml sterile water
    d. none of the above

40. A doctor wants to phone in a prescription for Percocet®

    a. you inform the doctor that the pharmacist must take the order.
    b. you ask the doctor if it is okay to use a generic.
    c. you inform the doctor that this drug cannot be phoned in.
    d. you take the order, but inform the pharmacist before filling.

41. Of the following group names, which one would be used for cough?

    a. antihelmintics
    b. antitussives
    c. antihistamines
    d. anticholinergics

Answers are at the end of the exam.

42. Tobrex® ophthalmic ung refers to

    a. an ointment used for the eye
    b. a solution used for the eye
    c. a topical ointment for external use only
    d. an ointment used for the ear

43. Suspending or thickening agents are added to suspensions to thicken the suspending medium and the sedimentation rate. Which of the following is not a Suspending agent?

    a. carboxymethylcellulose
    b. tragacanth
    c. acacia
    d. bentonite

44. Oral Polio Virus Vaccine (Poliovax®) should be stored in a temperature not to exceed 46 degrees Fahrenheit. What is this temperature in Centigrade? Use this formula: Centigrade = 5/9 (F° - 32°)

    a. 6.02 degrees C
    b. 7.84 degrees C
    c. 8.12 degrees C
    d. none of the above

45. You receive a prescription for amoxicillin 75 mg QID for ten days. How many mls of amoxicillin 250 mg /5ml do you need to fill this prescription to last the full ten days?

    a. 20 ml
    b. 40 ml
    c. 60 ml
    d. 100 ml

46. The doctor writes for aminophylline 125 mg po QID x 10 days. You only have the solution 250 mg/5 ml. How much would be needed for one dose?

    a. 1/4 teaspoonful
    b. 1/2 teaspoonful
    c. 3/4 teaspoonful
    d. 1 1/2 teaspoonful

Answers are at the end of the exam.

47. Of the following schedules, which one deals with drugs that have no medicinal use in the United States and have a high abuse potential?

    a. Schedule I
    b. Schedule II
    c. Schedule III
    d. Schedule IV

48. You receive a prescription for sertraline (Zoloft®) qd x 30 days. What is sertraline?

    a. antihypertensive
    b. anticonvulsant
    c. antidepressant
    d. antianginal

49. All aseptic manipulations in the the laminar flow hood should be performed at least

    a. four inches within the hood
    b. six inches within the hood
    c. eight inches within the hood
    d. twelve inches within the hood

50. Pharmacy technicians can perform their duties provided they

    a. check everything they do
    b. read all labels three times
    c. have all labels and products checked by a Pharmacist
    d. are certified

51. You receive an order for kaopectate 30 ml bid prn. How many tablespoonsful is one dose equal to?

    a. 5 tablespoons
    b. 3 tablespoons
    c. 2 tablespoons
    d. 1 tablespoon

52. Which of the following is a Schedule II Controlled Substance?

    a. diazepam
    b. meperidine
    c. pentazocine
    d. propoxyphene

Answers are at the end of the exam.

53. If the manufacturer's expiration date for a drug is 12/00, the drug is considered acceptable to dispense until which date?

    a. 12/01/00
    b. 12/31/00
    c. 11/30/00
    d. 1/01/01

54. The Roman numerals XLII is equivalent to:

    a. 42
    b. 62
    c. 92
    d. 402

55. A small volume intravenous bag specifically used to deliver medication is called an

    a. IV
    b. IVPB
    c. injection
    d. none of the above

56. How many days will the following prescription last?
    Prozac® 10mg #120   *Sig: 2 po BID*

    a. 20 days
    b. 30 days
    c. 45 days
    d. 60 days

57. The laminar flow hood should be left operating continuously. If it is turned off, it should not be used until it has been running for at least.

    a. ten minutes
    b. thirty minutes
    c. forty-five minutes
    d. sixty minutes

58. Which auxiliary label would you use for this particular sig: ii gtts AU bid?

    a. take with meals
    b. for the ear
    c. avoid sunlight
    d. for the eye

Answers are at the end of the exam.

59. A dose is written for 5 mg/kg every eight hours for one day. The adult to take this medication weighs 145 pounds. How much drug will be needed to fill this order?

   a. 765 mg
   b. 844 mg
   c. 989 mg
   d. 1254 mg

60. How much medication would be needed for the following order?
   prednisone 10 mg, one qid x 4 days, one tid x 2 days, one bid x 1 day, then stop

   a. 16
   b. 20
   c. 24
   d. 26

61. According to federal law, if an emergency prescription is received by telephone for a Schedule II drug, the prescriber must provide a written, signed prescription within

   a. 24 hours
   b. 36 hours
   c. 48 hours
   d. 72 hours

62. In which controlled substance schedule is Tylenol® No. 2 classified?

   a. Schedule I
   b. Schedule II
   c. Schedule III
   d. Schedule IV

63. Assuming that one pint is equal to 473 ml, how many pints can be found in one liter?

   a. 1.5 pints
   b. 2.1 pints
   c. 2.8 pints
   d. 3.1 pints

Answers are at the end of the exam.

64. Licensing and general professional oversight of pharmacists and pharmacies are carried out by

    a. colleges of pharmacy
    b. state board of pharmacy
    c. the American Pharmaceutical Association
    d. the United States Pharmacopeial Convention

65. Most unit-dose systems provide each patient with a storage bin in which can be found a supply of drugs for

    a. six hours
    b. eight hours
    c. twenty-four hours
    d. forty-eight hours

66. The first line of defense against infection/contamination of an IV product is

    a. antibiotics
    b. antiseptics
    c. disinfectants
    d. handwashing

67. The most widely used reference of an IV admixture program is the

    a. Handbook of Injectable Drugs
    b. Redbook
    c. Remington's
    d. Martindale's

68. Which of the following medications must be administered in a glass IV container?

    a. aminophylline
    b. dopamine
    c. nitroglycerin
    d. potassium

69. Preservative-free drugs must be used when drugs will be injected by which route of administration?

    a. intramuscular
    b. intrathecal
    c. intravenous
    d. subcutaneous

Answers are at the end of the exam.

70. The two parts of the syringe that should not be touched are

    a. the tip and needle
    b. the collar and barrel
    c. the tip and plunger
    d. the collar and plunger

71. The establishment of the Omnibus Budget Reconciliation Act (OBRA) in 1990, led to most states requiring

    a.) the use of pharmacy technicians
    b.) the counseling of patients by pharmacists
    c.) the enactment of the Controlled Substance Act
    d.) inventory management of each pharmacy setting

72. The first five digits of the National Drug Code (NDC) number identifies the

    a.) product
    b.) manufacturer
    c.) units
    d.) type of packaging

73. Sig or signa on a written prescription means

    a.) the strength of the medication ordered
    b.) the quantity of medication ordered
    c.) the directions for the medication ordered
    d.) the signature of the Practitioner writing the medication ordered

74. From the following directions how many tablets should be dispensed?
    2 tabs po qid x 2 days, then 1 tab po tid x 2 days, then ss po bid x 2 days, then dc

    a.) 22
    b.) 23
    c.) 24
    d.) none of the above

75. What should the last digit be of this DEA number?
    AB431762 __

    a.) one
    b.) three
    c.) five
    d.) seven

Answers are at the end of the exam.

76. Aminosyn is an amino acid often used in TPN orders to provide protein for cellular repair and growth. A physician writes an order for aminosyn 2.5% 500 ml. You have only aminosyn 8.5% 500 ml. How are you going to prepare this order using a sterile evacuated container?

    a.) add 320 ml of aminosyn 8.5% and qs with sterile water to 500 ml
    b.) add 147 ml of aminosyn 8.5% and qs with sterile water to 500 ml
    c.) add 124 ml of aminosyn 8.5% and qs with sterile water to 500 ml
    d.) add 74 ml of aminosyn 8.5% and qs with sterile water to 500 ml

77. You are to use 2.4 ml of diluent to reconstitute a vial of medication. What size of syringe should be used?

    a.) 20 ml
    b.) 10 ml
    c.) 5 ml
    d.) 3 ml

78. The use of isopropyl alcohol is important as a means to prevent contamination of an IV product. What should the minimum percent of isopropyl alcohol used be?

    a.) 50%
    b.) 70%
    c.) 90%
    d.) 100%

79. Most drugs and their metabolites are excreted by the

    a.) liver
    b.) kidneys
    c.) gall bladder
    d.) gastrointestinal tract

80. The percentage or fraction of the administered dose of a drug that actually reaches systemic circulation and the rate at which this occurs is the drugs

    a.) bioequivalence
    b.) bioavailability
    c.) biotransformation
    d.) therapeutic equivalence

Answers are at the end of the exam.

81. Most community pharmacies will have customers sign a log which records that the prescription was picked up. In most states signature logs are required for which of the following:

    a.) Medicaid prescriptions
    b.) third party prescriptions
    c.) Schedule V controlled prescriptions
    d.) all of the above

82. Zantac, Tagamet and Pepcid are H_2 blockers which are now available over-the-counter (OTC). What are these drugs used for?

    a. used as an antihistamine to alleviate runny nose
    b. used as an decongestant to unclog nasal passages
    c. used to inhibit stomach acid secretion
    d. used as an antacid in that it neutralizes stomach acid

83. A "hospital borne" infection is also known as a _____ infection.

    a. nosocomial
    b. infectious
    c. superinfection
    d. none of the above

84. Of the following drug recalls, which one is the most important in that all parties involved in the dispensing of a prescription (doctor, pharmacy and patient) must be notified due to the drugs potential or serious harm?

    a. Drug Recall I
    b. Drug Recall II
    c. Drug Recall III
    d. Drug Recall IV

85. Reconstitution with Ampicillin (Omnipen®) IVPB should be done with

    a. D5% Water
    b. 0.9% NaCl
    c. tap water
    d. vinegar

Answers are at the end of the exam.

86. A prescription for amoxicillin 250 mg #30 has a usual and customary price of $8.49. The acquisition cost of amoxicillin 250mg #30 is $2.02. What is the gross profit?

    a. $2.02
    b. $6.47
    c. 50%
    d. 1/3

87. A senior citizen is paying for a prescription for penicillin VK 250 mg #30. The usual and customary price is $8.49. However this patient qualifies for a 10% discount. How much will the patient pay?

    a. $8.49
    b. $6.99
    c. $8.39
    d. $7.64

88. NPH U-100 insulin contains 100 units of insulin per ml. The AWP for one 10 ml bottle of it is $18.45. The acquisition cost to the pharmacy for a 10 ml bottle is $16.70. The usual and customary price for one bottle of NPH U-100 insulin at that pharmacy is $14.99. If the pharmacy has an agreement with the third-party plan for reimbursement of 87% AWP or 100% U&C (whichever is less) + a $3.50 dispensing fee, what will be the total amount of the third-party claim?

    a. $18.49
    b. $19.55
    c. $20.20
    d. $21.95

89. A prescription is written for Septra Suspension 240 ml 1 teaspoonful h.s. + 1 refill. The insurance plan has a 34-day supply limitation. How many ml can be dispensed using the insurance plan guidelines?

    a. 120 ml
    b. 170 ml
    c. 240 ml
    d. 360 ml

Answers are at the end of the exam.

90. A prescription is written for Albuterol Inhaler: Dispense 2 inhalers of 17 gm, 2 puffs q.i.d. What is the days supply if there are 200 metered doses in each inhaler?

    a. 34
    b. 50
    c. 25
    d. 20

91. A prescription is written for Humulin N U-100 insulin 10 ml, 40 units daily. What is the days supply?

    a. 25
    b. 34
    c. 21
    d. 28

92. A prescription is written for Tetracycline HCl suspension 125 mg/5 ml compounded from capsules and a mixture of Ora-Plus 50% and Ora-Sweet 50%. How many capsules of Tetracycline 250 mg are needed to prepare 50 ml of this suspension?

    a. 5
    b. 10
    c. 15
    d. 20

93. Convert the Celsius temperature of 100 degrees into degrees Fahrenheit.

    a. 132
    b. 68
    c. 212
    d. 0

94. How many doses are in a 100 ml bottle of penicillin VK 250 mg/5 ml if each dose is 1/2 teaspoonful?

    a. 10
    b. 20
    c. 30
    d. 40

95. If 100 tablets contain 40,000 mg of ibuprofen, how many grains are in 500 tablets?

    a. 3,086
    b. 200,000
    c. 6,172
    d. 100,000

96. How many teaspoons equal 20 ml?

    a. 5
    b. 6
    c. 4
    d. 2

97. If a prescription reads: Aspirin 5gr, dispense 100 tablets, 1 tablet q 4-6h prn headache, what is the dose in milligrams?

    a. 650
    b. 750
    c. 100
    d. 325

98. How many gallons of Coca Cola fountain syrup are needed to package 150 bottles of 120 ml per bottle?

    a. 3
    b. 4
    c. 5
    d. 6

99. If a prescription reads: Amoxicillin 250 mg/5 ml, dispense 150 ml, 375 mg t.i.d. x 5d, what is the dose in household units?

    a. 1 teaspoonful
    b. 1 tablespoonful
    c. 1.5 teaspoonful
    d. 1.5 tablespoonful

100. How many ml are in 2 liters of normal saline?

    a. 200
    b. 2,000
    c. 0.2
    d. 0.002

Answers are at the end of the exam.

101. How many ml of KCl 2 mEq/ml are needed if the dose is 30 mEq?

   a. 5
   b. 10
   c. 15
   d. 30

102. How many ml of 25% dextrose are needed to prepare 500 ml of 40% dextrose if you are to prepare 40% dextrose from 25% dextrose and 60% dextrose?

   a. 214 ml
   b. 286 ml
   c. 200 ml
   d. 300 ml

103. If 1 liter is infused over 8 hours, what is the rate of infusion in ml/hr?

   a. 62.5
   b. 100
   c. 125
   d. 250

104. A patient weighs 121 pounds. What is the patient's weight in kg?

   a. 37
   b. 45
   c. 55
   d. 68

105. How many grams of sodium bicarbonate are needed to make 400 ml of a 1:1000 w/v solution?

   a. 0.2
   b. 0.4
   c. 0.8
   d. 1

106. Which of the following medications is associated with gradual discontinuation of therapy.

   a. Amoxil
   b. Sumycin
   c. Medrol
   d. Zovirax

Answers are at the end of the exam.

107. Alprozolam is a/an:

    a. narcotic
    b. barbiturate
    c. benzodiazepine
    d. stimulant

108. A medication to reduce fever is called a/an:

    a. antitussive
    b. antipyretic
    c. expectorant
    d. analgesic

109. What medication may cause an allergic reaction if a patient is allergic to penicillin and Ceclor?

    a. zithromycin
    b. doxycycline
    c. cefaclor
    d. amantadine

110. A prescription for Duragesic patches should be filed under which DEA schedule?

    a. Schedule I
    b. Schedule II
    c. Schedule III
    d. Schedule IV

111. Which of the following medications is most likely to be associated with photosensitivity?

    a. Bactrim
    b. Amoxil
    c. Suprax
    d. Cleocin

112. A pharmacist should be alerted about possible drug interactions when _____ and _____ are prescribed for the same patient.

    a. Zantac and Zocor
    b. Allopurinol and ibuprofen
    c. Darvocet N-100 and Dyazide
    d. Coumadin and Percodan

Answers are at the end of the exam.

113. Which of the following medications is classified in DEA Schedule III?

    a. Percodan
    b. Percocet
    c. Vicodin
    d. Valium

114. Which of the following medications is an antidiarrheal?

    a. propranolol
    b. famotidine
    c. methylphenidate
    d. loperamide

115. Vitamin A is a _____-soluble vitamin and Vitamin C is a _____ soluble vitamin.

    a. water, water
    b. fat, water
    c. fat, fat
    d. water, fat

116. Which of the following medications contains morphine?

    a. Demerol
    b. Dolophine
    c. MS Contin
    d. Mobigesic

117. If a medication is to be taken a.c., it should be taken

    a. in the morning
    b. around the clock
    c. after meals
    d. before meals

118. The federal agency associated with the Controlled Substances Act is

    a. ASHP
    b. DEA
    c. Treasury Department
    d. FDA

Answers are at the end of the exam.

119. The receipt of orders for Schedule III controlled substances can be documented on

    a. DEA Form 222
    b. Invoice/packing slip from wholesaler
    c. DEA Form 600
    d. FDA form 1210

120. Which DEA number fails the numerical check for DEA numbers?

    a. AK 6782329
    b. AB 3081421
    c. AG 1355672
    d. BS 3421234

121. An example of an H2 receptor blocker is:

    a. Pepcid
    b. Lomotil
    c. Chlor-Trimeton
    d. Prilosec

122. The directions "ii gtt o.u. q.i.d." indicate the medication is a/an

    a. otic
    b. ophthalmic
    c. oral
    d. ointment

123. _____ is an example of an anabolic steroid.

    a. methylprednisolone
    b. prednisone
    c. testosterone
    d. conjugated estrogens

124. Vasotec is a member of which of the following classes of drugs?

    a. antibiotic
    b. beta-blocker
    c. calcium channel blocker
    d. ACE inhibitor

Answers are at the end of the exam.

125. A pharmacist should be alerted if a patient is allergic to codeine and is prescribed

    a. Xanax
    b. Klonopin
    c. Tussi-Organidin
    d. Ritalin

ANSWERS TO PRACTICE EXAM

1.	b	45.	c	89.	b
2.	d	46.	b	90.	b
3.	a	47.	a	91.	a
4.	a	48.	c	92.	a
5.	b	49.	b	93.	c
6.	b	50.	c	94.	d
7.	b	51.	c	95.	a
8.	c	52.	b	96.	c
9.	b	53.	b	97.	d
10.	c	54.	a	98.	c
11.	c	55.	b	99.	c
12.	d	56.	b	100.	b
13.	d	57.	b	101.	c
14.	b	58.	b	102.	b
15.	c	59.	c	103.	c
16.	a	60.	c	104.	c
17.	d	61.	d	105.	b
18.	c	62.	d	106.	c
19.	d	63.	b	107.	c
20.	b	64.	b	108.	b
21.	a	65.	c	109.	c
22.	d	66.	d	110.	b
23.	c	67.	a	111.	a
24.	b	68.	c	112.	d
25.	c	69.	b	113.	c
26.	a	70.	a	114.	d
27.	c	71.	b	115.	b
28.	c	72.	b	116.	c
29.	c	73.	c	117.	d
30.	c	74.	c	118.	b
31.	a	75.	c	119.	b
32.	c	76.	b	120.	d
33.	a	77.	d	121.	a
34.	d	78.	b	122.	b
35.	b	79.	b	123.	c
36.	a	80.	b	124.	d
37.	a	81.	d	125.	c
38.	c	82.	c		
39.	b	83.	a		
40.	c	84.	a		
41.	b	85.	b		
42.	a	86.	b		
43.	c	87.	d		
44.	b	88.	a		

ANSWERS TO CHAPTER EXERCISES AND PROBLEMS

Chapter 1
p.4
1.   Shen Nung
2.   salicylic acid
3.   materia medica
4.   pharmaceutical
5.   panacea
6.   pharmacology
7.   Paracelcus
8.   data
9.   antitoxin
10. antibiotic
11. hormones
12. human genome
13. OBRA '90
14. formularies
15. managed care
p5.
1.   F
2.   F
3.   T
4.   F
5.   T
6.   T
7.   F
8.   F
9.   T
10. F

CHAPTER 2

p.8
1.   scope of practice
2.   personal inventory
3.   confidentiality
4.   patient welfare
5.   competent
6.   certification
7.   technicians
8.   professionals
9.   pharmacist
10. consulting
11. patient rights
12. detail oriented
13. continuing education
14. on-the-job training

p.9
1.   T
2.   F
3.   F
4.   T
5.   T
6.   F
7.   F
8.   T
9.   T
10. F

CHAPTER 3

p.14
1.   DEA number
2.   injunction
3.   placebo
4.   adverse effect
5.   legend drug
6.   negligence
7.   pediatric
8.   labeling
9.   "look-alike" regulation
10. liability
11. therapeutic
12. recall
13. controlled substance mark
14. NDC
p.15
1.   F
2.   F
3.   T
4.   T
5.   T
6.   F
7.   T
8.   T
9.   F
10. T
p.16
1.   Schedule II
2.   Schedule III
3.   Class III recall
4.   Schedule V

ANSWERS TO CHAPTER EXERCISES AND PROBLEMS

CHAPTER 3 CONT'D

5. Class II recall
6. Schedule I
7. Schedule IV
8. Class I recall

p.17
1. tight, light resistant
2. Endo Labs
3. Endocet
4. Oxycodone and Acetaminophen
5. tablets
6. oxycodone hydrochloride and aceta-minophen
7. C-II
8. room temperature
9. 01/00

CHAPTER 4

p.26
1. of each
2. before meals
3. right ear
4. morning
5. left ear
6. around the clock
7. each ear
8. to, up to
9. water
10. add water up to
11. distilled water
12. twice a day
13. with
14. capsules
15. give of such doses
16. dilute
17. dispense
18. divide
19. distilled water
20. elixir
21. fluid
22. gram
23. drop
24. hour
25. at bedtime
26. intramuscular
27. intravenous
28. intravenous push
29. injection
30. intravenous piggyback
31. liter
32. left
33. liquid
34. microgram
35. milliEquivalent
36. milligram
37. milliliter
38. normal saline
39. right eye
40. left eye
41. each eye
42. after meals
43. by mouth
44. as needed
45. each, every
46. every day
47. every hour
48. four times a day
49. a sufficient quantity
50. add sufficient quantity to make
51. without
52. subcutaneously
53. one-half
54. immediately
55. suppository
56. syrup
57. three times a day
58. tablets
59. tablespoon
60. topically
61. teaspoon
62. ointment
63. as directed

p.27
1. hypertension
2. thrombosis
3. phlebitis
4. arteriosclerosis
5. cardiomyopathy

6. endocrine
7. hyperlipidemia
8. hypothyroidism
9. somatic
10. anorexia
11. colitis
12. hepatitis
13. gastritis
14. dermatitis
15. subcutaneous
16. transdermal
17. hematoma
18. hemophilia
19. lymphoma
20. leukemia
21. tendinitis
22. neuralgia
23. osteoarthritis
24. endometriosis
25. vaginitis
26. prostatitis
27. bronchitis
28. pulmonary
29. sinusitis
30. cystitis
31. uremia
32. conjunctivitis

p.33
1. T
2. F
3. F
4. T
5. F
6. T
7. T
8. F
9. F
10. F

p.34
1. pneumonia, dehydration
2. penicillin allergy
3. every four hours by mouth
4. 2200 and 600 orders
5. 500 mg by mouth, every 12 hours
6. by mouth, each day
7. 8 hours

p.35
1. Prozac
2. 20 mg
3. capsules
4. by mouth
5. one capsule every day
6. 2
7. no

CHAPTER 5

p.32
1. prescription
2. extemporaneous compounding
3. protocols
4. signa
5. auxiliary label
6. medication orders
7. lookalikes
8. inscription
9. DAW
10. Rx
11. institutional labels
12. Schedule II, III, and IV auxiliary label
13. prescription number
14. DEA number

CHAPTER 6

p.38
1. 1.25
2. 0.005
3. 0.75
4. 0.67
5. 0.08
6. 0.425
7. 0.032
8. 0.8%
9. 50%
10. 4.2%
11. 12.5%
12. 7.5%
13. 40%
14. 2.5%

ANSWERS TO CHAPTER EXERCISES AND PROBLEMS

CHAPTER 6 CONT'D

Roman numerals:
15. IV
16. XLIX
17. LXII
18. CVIII
19. XXIV
20. XCVIII
21. XIV
22. 24
23. 104
24. 1200
25. 2 1/2
26. 18
27. 54

p.39, 42-43
1. 40
2. 21
3. 3.5
4. 2400 mg
5. 300 ml
6. 22.5
7. 720
8. 7.2 ml
9. 1.25 ml/min
10. 1.4
11. 360 ml
12. 500 ml 70% dextrose and 500 ml sterile water
13. 285 ml 70% dextrose and 715 ml sterile water
14. 250 ml 50% dextrose and 250 sterile water

p. 44
1.) aminosyn 500 ml
2.) dextrose 400 ml
3.) KCl 12 ml
4.) MVI 5 ml
5.) NaCl 5.45 ml
6.) sterile water 77.55

CHAPTER 7

p.49
1. F
2. T

3. F
4. T
5. F
6. T
7. T
8. T
9. F
10. F

p.50
1. local effect
2. systemic effect
3. degradation
4. adsorb
5. pH
6. inactive ingredients
7. enteric coated
8. water soluble
9. sublingual administration
10. hemorrhoid
11. parenteral
12. necrosis
13. sterile
14. intradermal injections
15. intravenous sites
16. aqueous
17. solvent
18. trauma
19. colloids
20. emulsions
21. intramuscular injection sites
22. subcutaneous injection sites
23. viscosity
24. biocompatibility
25. wheal
26. lacrimal gland
27. lacrimal canalicula
28. conjunctiva
29. transcorneal transport
30. nasal mucosa
31. nasal cavity
32. nasal inhaler
33. inspiration
34. metered dose inhalers
35. percutaneous
36. topical

37. hydrates
38. transdermal patches
39. Toxic Shock Syndrome
40. contraceptive
41. IUD

p.52
1. intraocular
2. intranasal
3. sublingual
4. inhalation
5. peroral
6. intravenous
7. vaginal
8. subcutaneous
9. intramuscular

p. 53
1. intradermal
2. subcutaneous
3. intravenous
4. intramuscular

Intramuscular
1. a
2. d
3. b
4. e
5. c

10. infusion
11. admixture
12. lyophilized
13. diluent
14. ready-to-mix
15. bevel
16. gauge
17. lumen
18. coring
19. membrane filter
20. depth filter
21. final filter
22. laminar flow
23. HEPA filter
24. biological safety hood
25. vial
26. ampule
27. sharps
28. equivalent weight
29. valence
30. molecular weight
31. ions
32. anhydrous
33. waters of hydration
34. osmosis
35. dialysis

CHAPTER 8

p.57
1. F
2. T
3. T
4. F
5. T
6. F

p.58
1. aseptic techniques
2. pyrogens
3. osmolality
4. isotonic
5. hypertonic
6. hypotonic
7. flow rate
8. heparin lock
9. piggybacks

CHAPTER 9

p.65
1. F
2. T
3. T
4. F
5. T
6. F
7. F
8. F
9. T
10. T
11. F
12. T

p.66
1. extemporaneous compounding
2. stability
3. anticipatory compounding

ANSWERS TO CHAPTER EXERCISES AND PROBLEMS

CHAPTER 9 CONT'D

4. calibrate
5. volumetric
6. arrest knob
7. meniscus
8. trituration
9. levigation
10. geometric dilution
11. sonication
12. solvent
13. saturated solution
14. supersaturated solution
15. syrup
16. Syrup USP
17. flocculating agents
18. elixir
19. suspending agent
20. miscible
21. immiscible
22. emulsifier
23. emulsion
24. water-in-oil
25. oil-in-water
26. hydrophilic emulsifier
27. lipophilic emulsifier
28. primary emulsion
29. mucilage
30. compression molding
31. fusion molding
32. "punch" method

CHAPTER 10

p.73
1. T
2. T
3. T
4. F
5. F
6. T
7. T
8. F
9. F
10. T
11. F

p.74
1. biopharmaceutics
2. site of action
3. receptor
4. selective action
5. agonists
6. antagonists
7. minimum effective concentration
8. onset of action
9. therapeutic window
10. disposition
11. passive diffusion
12. active transport
13. hydrophobic
14. hydrophilic
15. lipoidal
16. gastric emptying time
17. complex
18. protein binding
19. metabolite
20. enzyme
21. enzyme induction
22. enzyme inhibition
23. first pass metabolism
24. enterohepatic cycling
25. nephron
26. glomerular filtration
27. bioavailability
28. bioequivalence
29. pharmaceutical equivalents
30. pharmaceutical alternative
31. therapeutic equivalents

CHAPTER 11

p.78
1. hypersensitivity
2. anaphylactic shock
3. idiosyncrasy
4. hepatotoxicity
5. nephrotoxicity
6. carcinogenicity
7. teratogenicity
8. additive effects
9. synergism
10. interference

11. displacement
12. antidote
13. drug-diet interactions
14. hypothyroidism
15. hyperthyroidism
16. hepatic disease
17. cirrhosis
18. acute viral hepatitis

p.79
1. F
2. T
3. T
4. T
5. T
6. F
7. T
8. F
9. T
10. T

CHAPTER 12

p.82
1. primary literature
2. tertiary literature
3. abstracting services
4. Material Safety Data Sheets
5. secondary literature
6. American Hospital Formulary Service
7. Drug Facts and Comparisons
8. USP DI
9. Handbook on Injectable Drugs
10. World Wide Web
11. modem
12. browser
13. Internet service provider
14. URL

p.83
1. F
2. T
3. T
4. F
5. F
6. T
7. F
8. T

9. F
10. T
11. T

CHAPTER 13

p.86
1. open formulary
2. closed formulary
3. turnover
4. Schedule II substances
5. perpetual inventory
6. point of sale system
7. reorder points
8. order entry device
9. database
10. purchase order number
11. stock bottles
12. unit-dose
13. dispensing units

p.87
1. T
2. F
3. T
4. F
5. T
6. F
7. T
8. F
9. F
10. T

CHAPTER 14

p.90
1. pharmacy benefits managers
2. online adjudication
3. co-insurance
4. co-pay
5. dual co-pay
6. maximum allowable cost
7. U&C or UCR
8. HMO
9. POS
10. PPO
11. deductible
12. prescription drug benefit cards

CHAPTER 14 CONT'D

13. patient identification number
14. Medicare
15. Medicaid
16. Qualified Medicare Beneficiaries
17. workers' compensation
18. patient assistance programs
19. universal claim form

p.91
1. F
2. T
3. T
4. T
5. F
6. T
7. F
8. T

CHAPTER 15

p.94
1. OBRA '90
2. interpersonal skills
3. scope of practice
4. confidentiality
5. refrigeration
6. patient identification number
7. group number
8. signa
9. DEA number
10. safety caps
11. counting tray
12. shelf stickers
13. bar code
14. auxiliary labels
15. unit price

p.95
1. T
2. T
3. T
4. F
5. F
6. T
7. F
8. T
9. T

10. F
11. T

CHAPTER 16

p.100
1. Nurse Practitioner
2. Registered Nurse, R.N.
3. Licensed Practical Nurse, L.P.N.
4. unit dose
5. standing order
6. PRN order
7. STAT order
8. medication administration record (MAR)
9. code carts
10. centralized pharmacy system
11. inpatient pharmacy
12. decentralized pharmacy system
13. satellites
14. clean rooms
15. outpatient pharmacy
16. policy and procedure manual
17. distributive pharmacist
18. consultant pharmacist
19. automated dispensing system

p.101
1. F
2. F
3. T
4. T
5. F
6. T
7. T

CHAPTER 17

p.103
1. F
2. T
3. F
4. T
5. F
6. F
7. T
8. T

ANSWERS TO CHAPTER EXERCISES AND PROBLEMS

APPENDIX A

p.118

1. Proventil
2. Amoxil
3. Augmentin
4. Tenormin
5. Zithromax
6. Vancenase AQ
7. BuSpar
8. Fiorinal
9. Capoten
10. Carafate
11. Ceclor
12. Ceftin
13. Keflex
14. Tagamet
15. Biaxin
16. Bactrim
17. Valium
18. Voltaren
19. Lanoxin
20. Cardizem CD
21. Erythrocin
22. Desogen
23. Lo/Ovral 28
24. Pepcid
25. Prozac
26. Lasix
27. Vicodin
28. Advil
29. Humulin
30. Claritin
31. Ativan
32. Mevacor
33. Cycrin
34. Ritalin
35. Bactroban
36. Relafen
37. Naprosyn
38. Procardia
39. Axid
40. Prilosec
41. Daypro
42. Percocet
43. Dilantin
44. Pravachol
45. Deltasone
46. Zantac
47. Zocor
48. Imitrex
49. Nolvadex
50. Retin-A

p.120

1. insulin
2. antiemetics
3. gout
4. anti-hyperlipidemics
5. bactericidal
6. bacteriostatic
7. tuberculosis
8. dapsone
9. chemotherapy
10. Parkinson's Disease
11. cimetidine
12. nitrates
13. beta blockers
14. calcium channel blockers
15. isomer
16. inotropes
17. anemia
18. hematopoeitic drugs
19. anticoagulants
20. anabolic steroids
21. immunoglobulins
22. monoclonal antibodies
23. neuromuscular blockers
24. mydriatics
25. analgesic drugs
26. antipsychotics
27. sedatives
28. decongestants
29. antitussive
30. expectorants

KEY CONCEPTS INDEX

Page numbers indicate the start of the section in which the concept can be found.